A WORLD UNDIVIDED

A WORLD UNDIVIDED

A Quest for Better Healthcare
Beyond Geopolitics

JOSEPH SABA, MD

as told to MARIANA M. RODRIGUES

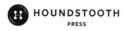

HOUNDSTOOTH
PRESS

A WORLD UNDIVIDED
A Quest for Better Healthcare Beyond Geopolitics

FIRST EDITION

ISBN   978-1-5445-3528-9   *Hardcover*
       978-1-5445-3527-2   *Paperback*
       978-1-5445-3526-5   *Ebook*

A Pascal

Vous êtes parti tôt même si vous avez résisté à votre maladie plus longtemps que prévu. J'ai fait ce que j'ai pu. Sans traitement c'était perdu ô combien je le regrette. Mais vous avez allumé en moi une flamme qui a sauvé bien d'autres et qui continue d'éclairer ma voie, et maintenant celle d'une nouvelle génération.

Reposez en paix.

***

To Pascal

You fought the disease longer than anyone could have expected, but still, you are gone too soon. I did all I could. Without treatment we lost the battle, and I regret it so much. But you lit a fire in me that saved many others. It continues to guide my journey and now the path of a whole new generation.

May you rest in peace.

CONTENTS

FOREWORD 9

PREFACE 13

1. TREATING A MAN, NOT A DISEASE...23

2. GRACE AND A NEW ERA OF GLOBALIZATION................................39

3. THE COUNTRY OF A THOUSAND HILLS...49

4. VIRUSES ARE SMART.. 61

5. BIRTH OF UNAIDS...77

6. TREATMENT CHANGES EVERYTHING...87

7. A CHICKEN AND EGG SITUATION 103

8. NEGOTIATING WITH THE BIG BAD WOLF 115

9. BRINGING TREATMENT TO AFRICA: THE STORY OF THE DRUG ACCESS INITIATIVE .. 127

10. IT'S POSSIBLE!...139

11. A STORY FOR THE AGES 149

12. A NEW GENERATION OF HEALTHCARE ACCESS 169

13. BREAKING BARRIERS 185

14. A NEW CHALLENGE..199

15. CAN WE REACH EVERYONE? 215

16. HEALTHCARE IN A FRAGMENTED WORLD..................................... 229

17. SACRIFICING UTOPIA FOR NECESSITY: A LESSON IN SUSTAINABILITY 245

18. MORE THAN AFFORDABILITY: CLOSING THE GAP OUTSIDE THE HOSPITAL 259

19. THE GREAT FACILITATOR 271

20. IT'S TIME WE MOVE FORWARD 283

ACKNOWLEDGMENTS.. 299

ABOUT THE AUTHOR 303

FOREWORD

By Michael Waldholz

I first met Dr. Joseph Saba in 1997 at a café along the Hudson River in New York City, near the offices of *The Wall Street Journal* where I had been a reporter for two decades covering healthcare and medical science. I recall our meeting so distinctly because it changed my reporting life in ways I couldn't have predicted. And it introduced me to Joseph, a disarmingly charming fellow who I was soon to learn was fierce in his commitment to shaking up long-entrenched and often failing global health policies.

Joseph was heading up an ambitious project for a newly formed World Health Organization agency, the Joint United Nations Programme on HIV/AIDS (UNAIDS). In our conversation, Joseph captivated me in describing the UNAIDS experiment to determine whether new and powerful, but also ultra-expensive, anti-HIV drugs could benefit people in Africa and other developing countries where HIV was spiraling out of control.

The disease was killing millions in these low-income regions, wreaking havoc on local economies and shredding the nations' social stability. Despite the obvious good intentions of the proposed UNAIDS venture, to my skeptical journalist's ears, given the drugs' high costs, it seemed like Saba and UNAIDS were tilting at windmills.

But it's a fool's game to underestimate what Joseph Saba can accomplish when he sets his mind to it. That is a lesson I learned over the following years of our professional and personal dealings. And it is the dramatic story Joseph shares in this book of his single-minded crusade to upend well-meaning but entrenched global healthcare practices that often fail the people in many low- and middle-income countries where these policies were designed to help.

Joseph can be persuasive. As evidence of that, soon after our conversation, I convinced my editors to let me tag along with Joseph and his small UNAIDS team to report firsthand on the AIDS crisis in Uganda, and whether Joseph's access plan was feasible. I'd never been to Africa, so of course, it seemed like an adventure I couldn't pass up. Little did I know AIDS in Africa would become a topic I would return to many times in the following years.

Reporting about developing world illnesses was not your typical *Journal* story. The previous year, a team of *WSJ* journalists that I led won a Pulitzer Prize for a year-long series of stories describing the discovery and impact of a remarkably potent triple-drug therapy that, for the first time, arrested the virus infection in those with the disease. I was eager to understand how that life-changing but expensive therapy would reach patients in areas of the world where they couldn't afford them.

During my time reporting on the story, I saw firsthand how deep the issues in the health system were. While I was skeptical of the solutions at first, it was obvious that we needed something different—for HIV patients, but also for other diseases and pandemics to come.

Clearly, an important goal of this book is to show how "out-of-box" ideas can be put into use. Joseph concedes that a good many of his efforts failed at first to meet initial objectives. But these setbacks led him and his teams to create other new solutions, many of which have become invaluable strategies that are being embraced throughout the global public health field.

Many lessons abound as Joseph, along with his co-author, Mariana Rodrigues, employ a good writer's narrative skills to show and not just tell, through their many adventures, how long-held beliefs and policies can be effectively overhauled. While the world has changed significantly since the HIV/AIDS pandemic, many of the same issues remain. An overhaul is needed indeed.

Given his forty years as a global health policy pioneer, Joseph ends his book with an out-of-the-box idea about globalizing the healthcare system. Not unexpectedly, his proposals may be controversial. Given his successes, however, I suggest his approach should be given serious consideration. For, as the book shows and as I learned myself, Joseph Saba has earned that right.

PREFACE

If you had told me a year earlier that I'd be carrying water buckets from the local well, I wouldn't have believed you. I grew up in a middle-class home in the Mazraa neighborhood of Beirut. My father, Jean, was an accountant, and my mother, Georgette, a secretary. Until 1975, I lived the typical life of a middle-class Lebanese sabi—or "boy" in Arabic. I attended the French Lycée school, spent half of my weekends running around the city with my friends, and spent the other half arguing with my younger sister Salma.

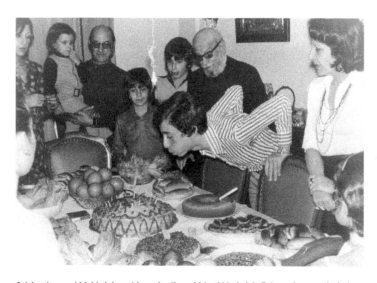

Celebrating my 14th birthday with my family and friend Mosbah in Beirut a few months before the start of the war.

On August 28, 1975, all of that changed. I was fourteen, and we were on vacation in Zahlé, inside Lebanon's Bekaa valley. For the adults, the war had started four months prior. For a week at a time—first in April, then in June—bombings were frequent and fighting roared across the country. Then things would go eerily quiet. As a kid, it took a while for the war to hit home. Until that day in August.

I remember feeling an uncomfortable tension in the air. One I never felt before. My parents were acting strange. Everywhere we went, shop owners and waiters talked about how anxious they were about the future. It's as if everyone knew something was coming, but none of us knew exactly what. As the situation worsened in Beirut, my parents worried about not being able to get back home. They eventually decided to cut our vacation short.

In August, the third round of hostilities began between Christian militias and armed Palestinian refugees, backed by Muslim militias. The tension between these groups had started a long time ago. In 1948, Palestinian citizens and fighters left Palestine (now Israel), seeking refuge in Lebanon and other neighboring countries. These tensions were amplified by religious and territorial agendas that inevitably grew into a civil war. Unlike the first two rounds of clashes that lasted no more than one or two weeks, this third round lasted for fifteen years and would eventually split Beirut and the rest of Lebanon into two warring factions of Christians and Muslims.

Afternoon bombings on civilian residential areas soon became a frequent occurrence. So did food and water shortages.

For the first year of the war, schools were closed. My best friend Mosbah and I had been classmates and neighbors since we were three years old. Now, at the age of fifteen, without a school to go to, we worked as electricians and renovated homes damaged by bombs. It's not how typical teenagers would spend their days, but Mosbah and I were products of the time. We did it because we liked feeling useful and, if you needed something during the war, you had to make it yourself. It was also a way to afford a few extra cakes from our favorite bakery. After all, though I didn't feel it then, we were still teenage boys.

We learned everything we knew about electricity from Dimitri, a family friend who had figured out a way to connect our block's powerlines to the neighboring street's. This got us a few extra hours each day of power—a luxury I didn't have to think about before the war.

Dimitri believed that in a time of crisis you can't wait for someone else to hand you a solution. You must take the reins and look outside the box. That rubbed off on me. When the light switch in my family's living room broke, sitting in the dark wasn't an option. I dismantled it piece by piece and eventually—nine hours later—fixed it.

As the years passed, we learned to live with war. I returned to school and my ongoing desire to understand how things worked became my greatest gift. My parents cultivated it. They did everything they could to make it possible for me and Salma to attend the best private schools and universities in Lebanon. It was this curiosity that led me to study medicine at St. Joseph University in Beirut. But it was the war that played a significant role in turning that curiosity into a lifelong inclination to not just accept things as they were. That inclination helped lead me into a career of learning, and ultimately to writing this book.

Three years into my medical studies, I had my first glimpse into what I thought could finally unite the country and bring the war to an end. It was that year that Bachir Gemayel was democratically elected president by both the Christian and Muslim members of parliament. The country seemed ready for change. We all hoped the dark days were over. But on September 14, 1982, before he could take office, he was assassinated. I heard the bomb that killed him from my desk at the university. It had become a familiar sound—as familiar as a bomb exploding can be, I suppose, but this one was strong and profound. I felt it deep in my body, like my heart was being torn. The president-elect had no chance to survive. Neither did our hopes.

During my medical residency in 1984, the fighting reached

another peak. I remember trying to triage hundreds of wounded patients at St. George Hospital with blood up to my ankles and spending night after night with little sleep trying to help injured patients as much as I could. One night, after a brutal attack by the pro-Syrian forces on the Lebanese army, I made a decision that would change my life forever.

That night, when working at the military hospital, I was asked to participate in the rescue of seriously injured Lebanese army soldiers still on the battlefield. These men were in such bad shape that they couldn't be transported to the hospital. For ten hours, we ran back and forth between the battleground and the ambulance where the supplies were stored and tried to administer intravenous painkillers to wounded soldiers in complete darkness. As the pro-Syrian forces encroached closer and closer to the presidential palace in Beirut, the situation seemed hopeless.

Suddenly, an incredible firewall of bombs hit the pro-Syrian forces. For nine hours, the American Battleship USS New Jersey continued its attack and made the pro-Syrians retreat back to their original positions. We were relieved, but we didn't understand what happened. It was no miracle nor providence. The Americans had come to the defense of the Lebanese army, setting an arbitrary red line five kilometers outside the Presidential Palace entrance gates that the pro-Syrians could not cross. By doing so, they showed who had the upper hand.

Everyone around me seemed happy, but I was deeply sad. The press often reported that Lebanon was being used as a pawn for geopolitical influence. Before that day, I didn't believe it, but now I saw it firsthand. I was on a battlefield, covered in the blood of wounded soldiers because I thought I could make a difference. It's why I stayed in Lebanon for so long. But we were just collateral damage. It was clear that the country had spiraled to a point where we were no longer in control of our fate.

Most people—at least those lucky enough to grow up without war or a revolution—don't think much about the systems that support our daily lives. We have trust that those systems—be it our electrical grid, our water supply, our hospitals, or government structures—will always be there to support us.

War taught me that the systems that support us are not forever. Eventually, they'll fail us—be it because of war, changing economic or political forces, or simply an inability to keep up with the evolving society in which we live. I learned early on in life that nothing is a given and nothing is to be taken for granted. If you want something, you need to ask for it, fight for it, and see it through. That realization took me to France to continue my medical education as an infectious disease physician and epidemiologist, then to Rwanda with the World Health Organization at the peak of the HIV/AIDS epidemic, and eventually to running a company focused on improving patient access to healthcare in parts of the world where it is needed most.

In those roles, I experienced firsthand what better healthcare can do for people and societies as a whole. Better healthcare gives us freedom to enjoy life as we want. It gives us more time to spend with our loved ones. It builds stronger, more resilient societies. Yet I also witnessed the direct repercussions of an antiquated, divided healthcare system overly dependent on the swaying tides of geopolitics. These obstacles continue to get in the way of real progress, and they are ultimately what led me to write this book.

When Al Razi conceived the first *bimaristan* (meaning "hospital" in Farsi) in Baghdad in the eighth century as a central hub for delivery of care, I doubt he ever imagined the concept would remain largely the same more than thirteen centuries later. Our population has grown many folds. Technology has evolved. Disease patterns have changed dramatically, and the availability of treatments that can be given at home (or at least outside a hospital) has opened the door to a new way of delivering care. Yet the healthcare system in place today has remained largely stagnant. Its inability to change became clear during the COVID-19 pandemic. We saw our healthcare infrastructure and systems fail before our eyes at a speed and scope none of us ever saw coming—including me. We saw governments haphazardly making decisions with no strategy nor vision, no unified scientific voice, doctors in overwhelmed hospitals having to prioritize one sick patient over another, and economic repercussions that will haunt us for decades.

In this book, you'll hear the term "healthcare systems" frequently. It's often used by those of us in public health to describe the institutions, people, and resources involved in delivering healthcare to people. It's not the sexiest term—doctors and scientists aren't typically known for their creativity in this area—but it's an important one to understand. Keeping people healthy requires many interconnected components working together.

Today's Healthcare System

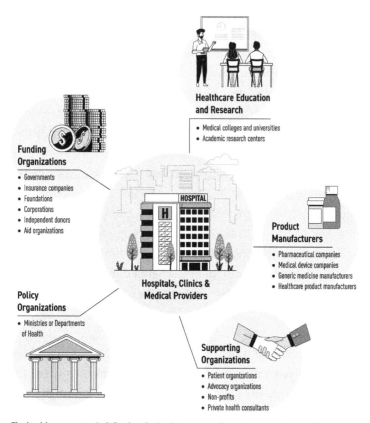

Healthcare Education and Research
- Medical colleges and universities
- Academic research centers

Funding Organizations
- Governments
- Insurance companies
- Foundations
- Corporations
- Independent donors
- Aid organizations

Product Manufacturers
- Pharmaceutical companies
- Medical device companies
- Generic medicine manufacturers
- Healthcare product manufacturers

Hospitals, Clinics & Medical Providers

Policy Organizations
- Ministries or Departments of Health

Supporting Organizations
- Patient organizations
- Advocacy organizations
- Non-profits
- Private health consultants

The healthcare system is defined as the institutions, people, and resources involved in delivering healthcare to people. Today's healthcare system is largely centered around local hospitals and health facilities.

To understand how we got here, we have to be willing to look back and learn. Healthcare doesn't work in a silo. It's a reflection of what is going on in the world. Starting in the 1980s, the HIV/AIDS pandemic was the first time in our modern history public health was put on the world stage, and hence where our story starts. *New York Times* reporter Larry Altman said:

As AIDS has become entrenched in the United States and elsewhere, a new generation has grown up with little if any knowledge of those dark early days. But they are worth recalling, as a cautionary tale about the effects of the bafflement and fear that can surround an unknown disease and as a reminder of the sweeping changes in medical practice that the epidemic has brought about. AIDS appeared shortly after the eradication of smallpox, which had renewed declarations of the demise of infectious diseases. As a result, public health leaders were not well prepared to deal with a newly recognized deadly disease.[1]

It's important to note that this book is not a history book. It does not intend to cover the full universe of global health milestones and happenings. Instead, my hope is that my own story of navigating the world of public health—however small it might be—will help shine some light on what a brighter future for healthcare can look like.

1   Lawrence K. Altman, "30 Years In, We Are Still Learning from AIDS," *New York Times*, May 30, 2011, https://www.nytimes.com/2011/05/31/health/31aids.html.

Chapter 1

TREATING A MAN, NOT A DISEASE

Pascal was thirty years old, just like me. He was a well-to-do business executive living in Paris with his wife and two young children. I've seen many patients in my life, but I'll always remember Pascal. Regardless of how sick he was, he was always in a neatly pressed suit, holding a shiny brown briefcase.

I saw him for the first time when he came into Bichat-Claude Bernard Hospital to be treated for pneumocystis pneumonia, a type of infection of the lungs in people with a weak immune system. That day, I had to tell him he was HIV positive.

Just four years earlier in Beirut, after that dreaded night trying to save soldiers near the Presidential Palace gates, I had made the decision to leave Lebanon to continue my medical education and practice in Paris. Eleven years in a war zone was enough. The fighting had escalated to the point where we were no longer in control of our fate. Treating soldier after soldier just to return them to the battlefields seemed pointless. I had become a doctor to help people. Instead, I was only putting a band-aid on a much bigger problem.

Looking out the plane window in July of 1986 at the country I loved so much, I felt a deep sadness. I knew I would never live there again. Beirut and all its complexities had made me who I was. But my experiences there also forced me to grow up sooner than most. Wartime Lebanon taught me that even the systems designed to support us and the leaders meant to protect us have limitations.

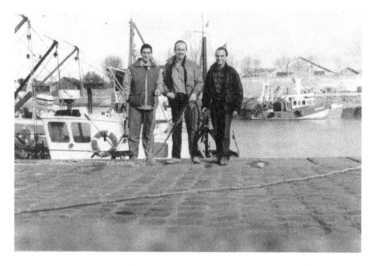

My lifelong friends Said and Joe posing in Normandy, France a few months after our arrival from Beirut.

My friends Joe and Said came to Paris with me, and our early days in France weren't easy. We worked days and nights—sometimes up to 100 hours each week. Much of our day work wasn't compensated, so we took jobs at night to earn our living. I didn't mind working around the clock and rebuilding my life from scratch. At least I was in control of my life again.

In France, I didn't hear bombs explode outside my bedroom window. I didn't need to worry about planning my day around the few hours of electricity. But what I didn't realize was that I had left one war zone for another. When I was in Beirut finishing medical school, I remember reading about HIV/AIDS in the papers. It felt like a disease of people very far away and very different from me. Now, suddenly, I was face to face with it.

When I first arrived in France in July 1986, I worked as an internal medicine clinician at Foch Hospital just outside of Paris. But my goal was to become an infectious disease physician. My fascination started with my first internship in the microbiology lab in Beirut. Back then, routine work focused on bacteria as our knowledge of viruses was limited. I learned how these living creatures, despite being nearly microscopic, were in fact so powerful, deadly, and above all, so adaptable. The more antibiotics we developed, the more they developed resistance to them.

In 1988, I began seeing HIV/AIDS patients at Claude Bernard Hospital, the hospital in Paris for the treatment of infectious diseases. Pascal was one of my first patients.

Around 100 years before I began making my rounds at Claude Bernard, the hospital had been inaugurated in preparation for the World's Fair in Paris—the same World's Fair that introduced the Eiffel Tower to the world. It was initially built to manage potential epidemics and infectious diseases that could result from the nearly 30 million people who came to the city that year. The hospital was built as over twenty separate pavilions to avoid cross-contamination, spread over 1km, with each pavilion dedicated to a specific infectious disease—measles, rubella, polio, tuberculosis. Once antibiotics were discovered, this concept was deemed less useful, and several attempts were made to close the hospital, thinking that infectious diseases were now under control.

Each time an attempt was made to close it, an epidemic would happen, forcing the Paris Hospitals Group and Ministry of Health to abandon their plans. Finally, in 1989, Claude Bernard was closed, and all staff and equipment were transferred to Bichat Hospital, a modern twenty-story hospital. The plans were implemented just as another outbreak was emerging—the HIV/AIDS pandemic.

The HIV/AIDS virus was first isolated and identified in 1983. It quickly became the subject of a contentious scientific squabble. Two teams, the National Cancer Institute in Bethesda, Maryland, led by Robert Gallo, and the Pasteur Institute in Paris, led by Luc Montagnier, debated over who discovered the virus, whose test for the virus was patented first, and whether one team had "appropriated" viral samples from the other. In 1991, Gallo finally admitted that the AIDS virus he had "discovered" really came from the Pasteur Institute. Luc Montagnier got the Nobel Prize for this discovery together with Francoise Barre-Sinousi, who was the first person to isolate the Human Immunodeficiency Virus (HIV) from the retroviruses family.

However, there is one part of this story that isn't often talked about. A brilliant infectious disease clinician who also happened to be a personal friend was the one who pointed Montagnier's team in the direction of the retrovirus family. In the late '70s, human T-cell lymphotropic virus (HTLV) was the first human retrovirus discovered. The HTLV-1 or HTLV-2 viruses infect white blood cells known as T cells and can cause aggressive leukemia and other neurological conditions. As he cared for patients with HIV, the physician found clinical similarities with HTLV-1 and told Montagnier's team to look for HTLV in their research. This is why the virus was initially named HTLV-3 (as HTLV-1 and 2 were already identified) before it was named HIV.

In 1985, American actor Rock Hudson became the first high-profile fatality from AIDS, drawing global attention to the disease. That same year, the first blood test for HIV became widely available. Global cases were estimated at 20,000, with every region of the world reporting at least one case of AIDS. Troubled by a growing number of cases, no public acknowledgment of the disease by politicians, and limited to no spending on AIDS research and treatment, activist groups began popping up across the US and Europe. These groups had a fundamental impact on the epidemic by refusing to accept the bureaucracy of the health system. They wanted immediate solutions, and their loud voices—which I would become the target of in the coming years—generated an unprecedented momentum that changed the international response to HIV/AIDS. More on that to come.

By 1989, the World Health Organization estimated 400,000 cases around the world—a 1,900 percent increase in four years, and a public health emergency at a level we hadn't seen in generations.

HIV is a virus that attacks the immune system, specifically CD4 cells (or T cells) that help the body fight a number of infections. Over time, HIV can destroy so many CD4 cells that the body can't fight infections and diseases, eventually leading to the most severe form of an HIV infection: acquired immunodeficiency syndrome, or AIDS. A person with AIDS is vulnerable to infections that are not typically contracted by healthy people. In AIDS patients, these infections often become life-threatening. The 36 million people who have died from HIV/AIDS since the start of the epidemic haven't died from the virus itself, but from the infections that occurred as a result of the body's weakened immune system.

Unlike many other infectious diseases, like COVID-19, malaria, and others, HIV/AIDS is a slow-moving disease. It's partly what makes it so horrible. HIV/AIDS patients need long-term care management and follow-up, like for a chronic disease, such as diabetes and high blood pressure. But infectious disease doctors weren't trained for that kind of disease profile, or for the non-medical complexities that come with treating a patient with a terminal disease for years and years.

As infectious disease physicians, we are taught to focus on prevention and treatment. But what if there is no treatment? What if the only medications available to help a patient feel slightly better cause severe side effects? How do you convince a patient to take such a medication day after day for years? What about the social and psychological implications of knowing that you have a disease that will—with 100 percent certainty—kill you? I had to find answers to many of these questions when treating Pascal.

Over the course of seven years, I saw him every month and helped him through what seemed like countless opportunistic infections. Each infection required a new medication, and there were many, many medications. Once the infection was resolved, I would try to take him off that medication or reduce the dosage. There was no medical or scientific reason why he needed to continue with that medication once the infection was resolved. But every time I took one away, he would deteriorate again.

Eventually, I decided to go against the medical guidelines and keep him on the medications that he told me made him feel better. Sometimes what is written in the medical guidelines or textbooks may apply broadly to the population, but not to one individual. Every person reacts differently.

Let me explain. Without the scientific standards captured in those books, modern medicine would never be where it is today. But there is a difference between rigor and rigidity. Rigor is the practice of maintaining strict consistency with certain predefined parameters. Rigidity, on the other hand, is an inability to be bent, forced out of shape, changed, or adapted. Rigor is critical to medicine; rigidity is detrimental and presumptuous. Why? Because it assumes that we know everything, when in fact every day we discover new patterns, new diseases, and new medicines. HIV/AIDS taught me this early in my career.

Sir William Osler, a Canadian physician credited with being the first to bring medical students out of the lecture hall for bedside clinical training, said, "The good physician treats the disease; the great physician treats the patient who has the disease." But that is easier said than done. For one simple reason: the way doctors and nurses are trained.

The basic structure of medical training hasn't changed in more than a hundred years. Medical education has traditionally been focused on science, as it remains today. Healthcare providers learn about the fundamentals of medicine, like anatomy, physiology, biophysics, and biochemistry. We also learn about diseases and their symptoms, and how to diagnose a patient. But all these lessons are taught in a silo, when in fact, there are many non-medical factors that affect a patient's condition, especially when it comes to managing a disease over a long period of time. Take disease stigma, for example, or the emotional challenges of being diagnosed with a terminal disease. Without addressing both of those factors, it is unlikely that a patient will fully benefit from the medication prescribed to them by their physician. Unfortunately, we providers are not taught to notice these things. We are taught to do the test, look at the numbers, and prescribe treatment—rather than think holistically.

Every patient has a story, specific needs, and challenges that affect how they respond to treatment. Sometimes, it is those nuances that make a difference between a patient living or dying. When I discussed this with other medical colleagues, we all nodded our heads and agreed. But living it through Pascal transformed the way I dealt with my patients completely.

The medical education system churns out thousands of brilliant physicians every year. But their brilliance is wasted trying to fit a square peg in a round hole. Many physicians today are trained to be rigid in their practices, relying exclusively on evidence-based medicine. In the majority of cases, this is both important and helpful. But when confronted with a new symptom or disease, it makes them unable to see outside the box. They are trained to dismiss the words *I don't know, maybe,* or *what if.* If a disease pattern or a sign is not documented and published, it must not exist.

That explains what happened one summer while I was on vacation. Pascal came into the hospital with a urinary tract infection (UTI). The doctors on call noticed his unconventional regimen and, one by one, removed all the medications deemed unnecessary. It made no sense, they said, and they were right. It didn't make sense according to the guidelines. A day later, he showed up at the hospital with a fever of 40 degrees Celsius (104 degrees Fahrenheit), where he stayed for three weeks until he was eventually put back on all his medications—as strange of a cocktail as it was. It's hard to say what role his unconventional medication regimen had in his disease progression, but who was I to take away a dying man's little remaining comfort?

HIV/AIDS made all of us working in the medical field take a long, hard look at the status quo, and whether the systems that had been traditionally set up to support patient care were effective. The disease presented a major challenge to hospitals and healthcare services as a whole. For one, it was new and not fully understood. Second, the disease is chronic and complex—affecting nearly every organ in the body and requiring ongoing medical care for a long period of time. Third, our response needed to go beyond medical interventions. Stigma and dire prognoses made psychological and social support critical. HIV/AIDS was a multidimensional disease that required a multidimensional and multi-sectoral response—but our providers and hospitals weren't set up for that.

Hospitals are not a modern invention. They were conceived in a time with challenges far different from our own. In the third century, the Romans set up the earliest concept of a hospital-like center. These units served more as patient relief dormitories, and little to no medical treatment was provided. It was between the eighth and tenth centuries, in the Persian and Arab worlds, that the Roman concept evolved to what we identify as a hospital today—a center of medical care. Hospitals were established from the notion that instead of a doctor going to see a patient individually in their homes, centralizing care in one place was a more efficient way to do it.

You'd think these early hospitals had nothing in common with our modern-day hospitals, but in fact, few things have changed. Certainly, the medical equipment and technologies have greatly improved. However, the hospital system, the way it works, and the way patients flow through the system are largely the same. A patient arrives, seeks medical care, gets treated, and leaves. There is often little to no relationship between the hospital and the patient outside these transactional medical acts, nor an effective system to support patients once they leave the hospital. Before the dawn of modern medicines that made it possible to treat many common diseases or ailments, this may have been sufficient because patients either healed or died. But by 1990, the world had changed significantly. For one, there were many more of us walking the Earth, and our population was getting older. We also had better medicines that kept people healthy, or at the very least, alive for longer. An epidemic was in full swing. Chronic diseases like diabetes, hypertension, and heart disease were also on the rise. More patients needed treatment that would be administered regularly and last for years, making it virtually impossible to keep care centralized to the walls of a hospital building. For these, among many other reasons, hospitals in many countries were quickly overwhelmed by HIV/AIDS.

In November 1991, a *New York Times* article reported on the toll of HIV on New York City's largest municipal hospital, Kings County Hospital Center in Brooklyn: "Patients come in sicker and stay longer. They are emotionally needier and ask more frequently whether they are going to die. Some complain of discriminatory treatment …100–110 patients—about 10 percent of the hospital's in-patient population—suffer from an AIDS-related condition at any given time. In some wards these patients take up more than 80 percent of the beds."[2]

This example illustrates the problem hospitals and clinics faced around the world. They were overloaded with patients who needed more than medication. They needed to be listened to. They were stigmatized, many had lost their jobs as a result of their diagnosis, and others were rejected by their families and friends. Finding beds for our HIV/AIDS patients required delicate negotiations and difficult decisions. We were constantly on the search for non-AIDS patients whose conditions warranted a discharge in order to free up a bed.

Cities and hospitals around the world looked for ways to triage the growing deluge of HIV cases. In France, we established a general practitioners (GPs) network to keep open contact with patients' GPs and trained them on HIV management to help reduce the frequency of hospital visits. We also progressively introduced psychological and social support services. In my hospital, the psychologist, Zohra, took care of patients as if they were her family. She frequently came by to discuss patients' problems and apprehensions they didn't feel comfortable sharing with us physicians. Nadine, the social assistant,

2   Mireya Navarro, "Treating AIDS: One Hospital's Struggle - A Special Report; Epidemic Changes All at Inner-City Medical Center," *New York Times*, November 11, 1991, https://www.nytimes.com/1991/11/11/nyregion/treating-aids-one-hospital-s-struggle-special-report-epidemic-changes-all-inner.html.

helped patients with completing reimbursement paperwork and securing unemployment benefits when they lost their jobs. Dr. Melchior and Celine, both nutritionists, followed the patients closely and prescribed vitamins and supplements. Activists, who themselves were living with HIV/AIDS, met with patients every week. They provided psychological counseling and held art and theater workshops. Patients loved it and felt energized. These weren't traditional medical interventions, but there was little that existing medicines could do for AIDS patients at that point. We had to find other ways.

Pascal was in frequent touch with Zohra and Celine. I don't think we would have been able to keep him alive as long as we did without these non-medical interventions. As a physician, I have no doubt that the medical response is the core of any patient care. Yet I learned over the years that while it is necessary and indispensable, medical care is often not sufficient on its own. This is not what I was taught in medical school. This is what patients taught me and continue to teach me every day.

Despite the challenges of the time, we quickly learned that multidimensional interventions work. An average AIDS patient in the late '80s lived approximately three to five years after diagnosis. With all the support we provided, we managed to increase the survival time for many of our patients and help them to live their remaining years more comfortably.

We were able to keep Pascal with us for seven years before he passed away at the age of thirty-seven. I had grown close to him over those years. I remember a day, looking out a window of the intensive care unit, seeing the Eiffel Tower illuminated. "How far I've come," I thought. "All the way from Lebanon."

But one thing hadn't changed. I was still surrounded by death and hopelessness. Seeing Pascal deteriorate before my eyes, it was horrible to not have anything more to offer him. We were close in age and mind. He could have been my personal friend. I certainly felt so, and I believe he did too. We used to talk about many things together, not just his medical condition. When his disease advanced, I had to advise him to plan his succession. It was quite a difficult moment for him, and for me. As hard as it was, I felt it was my commitment to him as my patient. I was essentially telling him to prepare himself for death—and there was nothing I could do about it. I felt helpless.

If the war in Lebanon taught me anything, it was not to give up when there is hope. The French government had recently formed the National Agency for AIDS Research (ANRS), which brought together experts from around the country to conduct research to improve the treatment of HIV and its co-infections. My boss at Claude Bernard Hospital gave me the responsibility of managing and monitoring one of the ANRS's first trials: ANRS 004. The trial focused on the treatment of pneumocystis pneumonia, one of the first opportunistic infections to occur in AIDS patients. It was there that I found hope. Thanks to my boss, I learned that research wasn't just data on a page, but a tool for improving patients' lives.

I had just finished my master's degree in statistics, and one of my professors was a high-profile statistics scientist who developed a novel trial methodology called "pragmatic trials" aimed at research in real-world situations. The methodology is slightly different from traditional clinical trials that look at an experimental "ideal" situation rather than real life. The ANRS 004 trial was a pragmatic trial. It analyzed different treatment strategies in real-world situations versus the best possible scenario, as is typically done in clinical trials. This trial methodology would prove to be increasingly useful in HIV/AIDS research in the years to come as traditional clinical trial methodologies were often difficult to implement in low- and middle-income country settings. Working on ANRS 004, I learned to understand research results and read between the lines. How useful is a statistical result if it has minimal clinical application in the real world? Like medicine, statistics is not black and white. You have to be pragmatic and use your common sense to interpret the results.

Research gave me hope while also opening new horizons in my career. It allowed me to visit clinical trial centers to better understand how they operate and collaborate with fellow researchers in the US and Europe, and present at medical conferences. I was happy, full of energy, and tireless. I was in the heart of the action. I could make a difference again.

I didn't realize it then, but the ANRS 004 trial was one of the first of what was to become a growing movement of collaborative initiatives by the scientific community against HIV/AIDS, driven by the tumultuous yet promising geopolitical shifts of the late '80s and early '90s.

The '80s saw the collapse of traditional communism and the end of the Cold War, a period of geopolitical tension between the Soviet Union and the United States and their respective allies after World War II. Europe was carved up by the Soviet Union and its former Western allies, and the Soviets gradually erected an "Iron Curtain" splitting the East from the West. Defeated, Germany was divided up by the occupying powers—the US,

UK, France, and the USSR—with the eastern part occupied by the Soviets. East Germany, officially known as the German Democratic Republic, became the Soviet Union's foothold in Western Europe. But Berlin was split four ways, with British, French, and American zones in the west of the city and a Soviet zone in the east. West Berlin became an island surrounded by communist East Germany. The Berlin Wall was eventually built in 1961 because East Berlin was hemorrhaging citizens to its western rivals.

By the mid-1980s, the Soviet Union faced significant economic problems and major food shortages. When a nuclear reactor at the Chernobyl power station in Ukraine exploded in April 1986, it brought to light the run-down infrastructure of the USSR and marked a symbolic moment in the impending collapse of the Communist Bloc. Cracks in the Soviet Bloc had already started to appear in the 1980s with a series of protests from Hungary to Poland to Czechoslovakia. But it was the fall of the Berlin Wall, the very symbol of communist repression, which ultimately marked the end of this divisive era.

On November 9, 1989, five days after half a million people gathered in East Berlin in a mass protest, a spokesman for East Berlin's Communist Party announced citizens of East Germany were free to cross the country's borders. East German leaders had tried to calm mounting protests by loosening the borders, making travel easier for their citizens. They had not intended to open the border up completely. The changes were meant to be fairly minor—but the way they were delivered had major consequences. Notes about the new rules were handed to the spokesman, Günter Schabowski, who had no time to read them before his regular press conference. "Private travel outside the country can now be applied for without prerequisites," he said. Almost immediately, Berliners began slamming the wall with axes and sledgehammers. By nightfall, the celebration turned into what one observer called "the greatest street party in the history of the world." East and West Germany would reunite one year later.

The fall of the Berlin wall and the official end of the Cold War came at a time when technology began to take center stage. The world was introduced to the internet in 1983 for the first time, and the likes of Microsoft, IBM, Intel, and Apple began to sell smaller, cheaper computers that changed technology from an industrial good to one available for personal consumption.

The world was entering a new era—one marked by newfound hope and global cooperation and driven by innovation. That hope made its way to public health. AIDS had become the first illness debated in the United Nations (UN) General Assembly. No longer paralyzed by the Cold War, the UN was becoming increasingly prominent. The world was starting to pay attention. Perhaps soon, patients like Pascal would no longer have to die.

Chapter 2

GRACE AND
A NEW ERA OF
GLOBALIZATION

In many ways, the beginning of the HIV/AIDS crisis in the early- to mid- '80s was similar to what we saw in the early days of the COVID-19 pandemic. Countries struggled to contain cases. While they were all facing the same problem, there was little collaboration. Instead, as HIV/AIDS cases surged, the nations of the world were driven by Cold War-era urges to protect their turf and erect a slew of unnecessary borders—geographic, social, and economic.

Even as governments attempted to act alone, they were all using the same data to guide their decisions. That rationale would say similar decisions could be expected, right? Not so. Leaders sought to differentiate their "sovereign" nation from others and often charted courses meant to show the uniqueness of their country. Some countries chose to pretend the HIV/AIDS epidemic was not a serious issue at all. Others locked down their countries and forbade people with the virus to enter.

There is no doubt that the HIV/AIDS epidemic could have been better contained with a quicker, proactive, and more coordinated response from the world's leaders. Government bureaucracies slowed down and complicated the public health response, contributing to insufficient funds directed toward AIDS research and limiting support at a time when the world needed it most. Instead, many displayed a staggering incompetence or apathy. There were many reasons for this. None of them were valid. There were biases resulting from a disease that at first was perceived as largely affecting already stigmatized communities, such as gay men, sex workers, drug users, and migrants. There were efforts to hide the crisis for fear of potential political implications and later because politicians falsely believed that the HIV epidemic was mostly a concern of lower-income countries with less developed healthcare systems.

These, among other barriers, prevented the world from responding to HIV/AIDS as it should have. We are used to thinking of barriers as physical divisions—a geographic border outlining the area a particular governing body controls. But religion, economics, and our political ideals are barriers too. In an era in which globalization was increasing rapidly, these imaginary barriers did little to contain a virus. Instead, they fueled the epidemic and opened the world's eyes to severe double standards in healthcare between the haves and have-nots. The idea of acting "within our borders" cannot work on a borderless virus. Global challenges need global responses. The HIV/AIDS epidemic soon became everyone's problem. For the first time in our modern society, we were facing a public health issue of global proportions. It was a pandemic.

Thankfully, the end of the Cold War gave way to more international collaboration and scientific progress in AIDS research and brought new hope to what, at the time, seemed like an unsolvable problem. The paralysis that had plagued the world for more than forty years following World War II came crashing down, along with the Berlin Wall that divided us until that fateful November day.

The fall of the Berlin Wall was a pivotal event in world history for many reasons. It marked not only the dismantling of the Iron Curtain, but also the start of the collapse of communism in Eastern and Central Europe, which, in turn, triggered a series of world events that would affect every aspect of our livelihood, from the economy to national security, to—you guessed it—healthcare.

Allow me to explain.

Mikhail Gorbachev, who was president of the Union of Soviet Socialist Republics (USSR) in 1988, knew that radical reforms were needed to sustain its economic and social model during the Cold War. Gorbachev faced powerful critics from conservatives inside the Communist Party and reformists like Boris Yeltsin, president of Russia, who thought he was not doing enough to stop the likely collapse of the Soviet Union. In December of 1991, Gorbachev resigned, leaving Yeltsin as president of the newly independent Russian state.

Just weeks after the dissolution of the Soviet Union, US President George H.W. Bush and Boris Yeltsin met at Camp David to formally declare the end of the Cold War, which triggered a series of world events, under what became known as the "new world order." The term "new world order" was used by Bush in a joint session of the US Congress to define the post–Cold War era and the spirit of cooperation that he hoped would follow:

> We stand today at a unique and extraordinary moment. The crisis in the Persian Gulf, as grave as it is, also offers a rare opportunity to move toward an historic period of cooperation. Out of these troubled times, our fifth objective—a new world order—can emerge: a new era—freer from the threat of terror, stronger in the pursuit of justice, and more secure in the quest for peace. An era in which the nations of the world, East and West, North and South, can prosper and live in harmony. A hundred generations have searched for this elusive path to peace, while a thousand wars raged across the span of human endeavor. Today that new world is struggling to be born, a world quite different from the one we've known. A world where the rule of law supplants the rule of the jungle. A world in which nations recognize the shared responsibility for freedom and justice. A world where the strong respect the rights of the weak. This is the vision that I shared with President Gorbachev in Helsinki. He and other leaders from Europe, the Gulf, and around the world understand that how we manage this crisis today could shape the future for generations to come.[3]

Collaborative military interventions driven by the "new world order" during the Gulf War and Balkan Wars gave rise to a concept called the "right to intervene." Promoted by Ber-

---

3   "Public Papers: Address Before a Joint Session of the Congress on the Persian Gulf Congress and the Federal Budget Deficit," George H. W. Bush Presidential Library & Museum, September 11, 1990, https://bush41library.tamu.edu/archives/public-papers/2217.

nard Kouchner, a prominent French diplomat, politician, and co-founder of Médecins Sans Frontières (Doctors without Borders), the concept was founded on the idea that countries had a moral obligation to interrupt the national sovereignty of other nations to defend human rights. Kouchner believed that human rights—not states—should rule the world.

Supporters of the concept saw the growing humanitarian sentiments of the '90s as necessary action in the face of human rights abuses. To its detractors, it was viewed as an excuse for military intervention. In other words, "humanitarian imperialism." Its frequent use following the end of the Cold War suggested to many that a new norm of military humanitarian intervention was emerging in international politics.

Around the same time, the war in Lebanon that started when I was fourteen years old finally ended. I never thought I'd live to see the end of that conflict. But here we were. We were entering an entirely new era. One by one, the geo-political and humanitarian developments of the early '90s would shape generations to come and serve as key drivers of progress over the following thirty years.

What does this all have to do with healthcare? The way we address healthcare challenges is a reflection of what is happening in the world. Eventually, the implications of our newly globalized world knocked on my door.

* * *

In the late '80s, most of my HIV/AIDS patients were homosexual and bisexual men. Then I began to see more IV drug users.

Eventually, in the early '90s, Africans started coming through our doors.

It was 1992 when I first met Grace, a young African diplomat living in Paris. She had come to the hospital with her brother, who was newly diagnosed with HIV and still asymptomatic.

One day the phone rang in my office. It was Grace and she wanted to come in for an urgent appointment. Her boyfriend had flown in the day before and she explained to me that while they typically used condoms, this time they didn't. She asked him to get tested, and he tested HIV positive. She was worried she had been infected herself.

We tested her the day after to see if she was positive, already knowing that it typically takes ten days to a month for a patient to develop the antibodies that would result in a positive test. Grace's first test came back negative, and we all breathed a sigh of relief.

A month later, when it came time to get the results of her second test, we weren't so lucky. I opened Grace's file to prepare for the consultation and I froze. The test had come back positive. She was only a couple of years younger than me, highly educated, smart, with a bright future ahead of her. But the virus paid no attention. The virus doesn't care how wealthy you are, what country you come from, your race, your profession, or your sexual orientation.

"Because of one night, my life will never be the same," Grace told me in shock.

Knowing that her life expectancy dropped to ten years if we

didn't find a treatment, I nodded sadly. As a young doctor coming to grips myself with the ferocity of the HIV/AIDS epidemic, what could I possibly have said to make this okay?

I wanted to do more. What could I do to stop the spread of this disease? Every day in the hospital, I was helping patients. It was a critically important job. But it was limited.

At home, I repeatedly shared my need and rage to do more with my wife, Marie-Helene. Tired of hearing about my frustrations, she encouraged me to look beyond clinical care and consider entering the field of international public health. As a doctor, my view of healthcare at that time was one strictly based on the interactions between me and the patient. Going into the world of international public health would require a much broader view of the factors driving the overall health of an entire population. It sounded like just what I was looking for.

Never one to think small, I began planning how I could get a position at the World Health Organization (WHO). My only connection—albeit a loose one—was a UN translator who was an old friend of mine. She put me in touch with another Lebanese doctor who worked at WHO. I managed to book a meeting with him in Geneva, Switzerland, where the WHO headquarters is located.

The meeting went as expected—"thanks for your interest, but there are no positions available." He made it clear to me that working at WHO wasn't like any other job. Most employees had grown up in the global public health world, which—I didn't realize then—was rather small and insular. You couldn't just walk in from the street and ask for a job.

But taking no for an answer is not in my book. I went back time and time again until I was able to get a meeting with the then head of the HIV vaccine unit. After a few meetings, he told me there was a position in Rwanda for HIV vaccine research sponsored by the French government. They needed someone who spoke French, and although I'd love to say that it was my experience that got me the opportunity, the reality was that I was in the right place at the right time. If I could get approval from the French government for the job, it was mine, he said.

I immediately went to see my boss, who was Head of Infectious Diseases at Claude-Bernard Hospital and my mentor. He told me the position would be overseen by the ANRS, the same organization that supported the ANRS 004 trial I managed. He called the Head of ANRS, who knew me through my previous work in their clinical trials, and who supported my candidacy immediately. A few weeks later, I was offered the position to prepare an open cohort for a potential HIV vaccine trial in Rwanda.

In hindsight, I don't know what I was thinking. I had little to no public health experience. I was only thirty-two years old (most at WHO were over fifty with thirty years of experience under their belts). I just went for it. For better or worse, I've always felt that I could figure it out.

The role opened my eyes to an entirely new world and set the wheels in motion for what would become my lifelong calling to improve access to healthcare.

I am eternally thankful for Grace for having opened my eyes. And of course, to my wife for encouraging me to pursue a new direction.

In the end, unlike Pascal, Grace was one of the lucky ones. By the time she was diagnosed, she didn't have to wait long to receive antiretrovirals (ARVs). She also had the means to afford them at a time when ARVs, despite being available, were beyond reach for 80 percent of the world. Grace became a family friend and has since gone on to work for some of the largest public health organizations in the world. I have no doubt that her unexpected diagnosis that afternoon almost thirty years ago in my office drove her decision to enter the world of public health. Certainly, "because of one night, her life was never the same again."

Chapter 3

THE COUNTRY OF A THOUSAND HILLS

In April 1993, I boarded my first flight to the African continent, headed to Rwanda. Rwanda is known as the country of a thousand hills. I opened my window as we landed on a small runway, so tiny it felt like it could barely hold the equally tiny plane we were in. Beyond this strip of dirt, however, it was astounding: the lush, green earth rose and fell as far as I could see. Kigali, the capital and largest city in Rwanda, sits on top of one of these hills, 5,151 feet above sea level. It was a statistic that became very real to me when I tried to play tennis my first week and couldn't last more than fifteen minutes.

My goal was to spend the first month before my family arrived getting the necessary partners together and securing funding— but there was little precedent for how to go about doing that and few systems in place to support us. I didn't know what to expect, and in hindsight, I had little sense of the challenges ahead. I had to figure it out.

There is something about Africa that is unlike any other place on Earth. There is a sense of space and freedom that makes you feel alive and like anything is possible. I know that many Africans don't feel the same. But for those of us coming from major, over-populated cities in Europe, the Middle East, or Asia, we were accustomed to a life burdened with rigorous norms and regulations. Every decision I made in Beirut or Paris was clouded by bureaucracy, societal expectations, and rules for what is and is not acceptable. Some might say that these norms are necessary to regulate crowded cities with millions of people—and they are, to a certain extent. But when they go too far, a society can become rigid and less adaptable. That includes the healthcare system needed to keep that society healthy, which can become so regulated that innovation becomes either a distant prospect or an unachievable goal. Rwanda was uncharted territory—at least it was for me. With little infrastructure came freedom and the opportunity to do more, a lot more. It was both overwhelming and exciting. Thankfully, I had some wonderful Rwandans and expats to show me the ropes.

As a UN official, I was assigned a Rwandan counterpart by the Rwandan government named Jacques. Jacques opened many doors for me when I first arrived. He taught me much of what I know about Rwanda, its culture, and its people. Over my first few months in the country, we became close. I was also part-nered with Joel, a French researcher seconded by the French Ministry of Cooperation, an organization already in Rwanda running a study on pregnant women and HIV/AIDS. Joel helped me with my move and to navigate Rwanda. He remains one of my best friends to this day.

When Marie-Helene and my boys, Jean Noel and Eliott, arrived in May, we moved into our home high above the beautiful hills of Kigali and began learning the culture. For example, we never had a cook or a driver before, and didn't intend to start now. We were used to being and preferred to remain autonomous. But we learned that Rwandans saw expats coming into the country as a job opportunity, and denying them this opportunity would not be a good way to start. Before we knew it, Wadi became our dedicated cook, Joseph our guard, Francois our eager gardener (who seemed to enjoy pushing Eliott around in a toy car perhaps more than gardening), and Lilian, our beloved babysitter who loved our boys like her own. There weren't many blond children in Rwanda, and Lillian took every opportunity to show them off. From early on, I loved the country and its people.

My job was to prepare and oversee open cohorts mostly in Kigali, with one site in Butare, for a potential HIV vaccine trial, while studying the effectiveness of different follow-up and prevention methods. What that meant was that I was responsible for setting up groups of people susceptible to HIV infection, following them closely for a period of time (three years in our case), and providing education and preventive measures to hopefully prevent them from getting the disease. If cohort participants got infected, they would exit the cohort and join a treatment clinical study. For those who did not get infected, when the vaccine became ready for a clinical trial, this group would receive the investigational vaccine as study participants. Clinical trials were not typically done in Africa, and these cohorts were designed to help us better understand what to expect on the ground so we could be as effective as possible once the trials started.

In a closed cohort, no additional subjects are added after initial recruitment, causing the number of subjects to decline because of infection or death. As the pool shrinks, so does the incidence rate, making it difficult to assess whether a vaccination is effective or there are simply fewer infections. In contrast, an open cohort is dynamic, meaning that members can leave or be added over time. We chose to use an open cohort that is constantly resupplied with new patients so we could keep a steady incidence rate. When the time came to vaccinate, if we saw a drop in infection, we could more easily attribute it to the vaccine.

I collaborated with research groups to oversee several open cohorts—including pregnant women, discordant couples (or couples in which one person is HIV-negative and the other is not), sex workers, and people enrolled in select voluntary counseling and testing (VCT) centers. Our goal was to recruit participants who were representative of the general population, but also those most vulnerable to infection, and to closely follow them while providing education and prevention tools. These cohorts—funded by organizations in the US and Europe—were already in place in Rwanda, but were not previously being used for the purpose of eventual vaccination. We chose to use these existing cohorts to get us up and running as quickly as possible—working under the expectation that the vaccine would soon be ready for clinical trials.

But identifying the cohorts was only the beginning. We also had to build systems that would allow us to follow up with these patients and reach them for prevention interventions. Additionally, we had to create mechanisms to support patients who would become infected despite our prevention methods.

In many countries, we could rely on clinics and hospitals to report much of this to us, but that wasn't the case in Rwanda at this time. While clinics and hospitals existed across the country, they weren't linked to each other and there were no patient files. Instead, we embarked on a sometimes tedious though mostly effective journey of personal follow-up. We made thousands of phone calls, and when that didn't work, we went to their houses. The value of everything we were doing was tied to our ability to follow patients, and we had to make it happen, no matter what it took.

Prevention was easier said than done. During my first few days on the job, I expected that prevention would be an easy sell. Why wouldn't you want to prevent a disease that could kill you? Instead, what I found was that many people were not as concerned as I expected, especially men. Sickness was often seen as a sign of weakness for men, resulting in a reluctance to seek care. There was also evidence men saw testing as something that would make public the sexual behaviors they wanted to keep secret. Plus, they were much less likely to seek care without the availability of treatment. I witnessed similar issues across genders, ages, and socioeconomic classes. It was as if trying to prevent HIV was almost as bad as having HIV. Wearing a condom, for example, was seen by some as an admittance of their risky, taboo sexual behavior. Instead, denying the risk and going forward with business as usual was a more comfortable, palatable option—at least until they became infected. You may have seen humanity's similar reluctance toward preventative behavior during COVID-19.

By the time I was in Rwanda, that new class of drugs called antiretrovirals, or ARVs—the one that Grace was able to use— was already available to HIV/AIDS patients in richer countries in the US and Europe. These early medications came with limited effectiveness and unpleasant side effects, but at least they were something. In Africa, we had nothing. Even the vaccines we were preparing for were only in the early research stages. We did our best to manage opportunistic infections, which are infections that occur more often or are more severe in people with weakened immune systems, but that required early diagnosis and close disease management—both of which were hard to implement in Africa and other low- to middle-income countries. That is why the early public health battle against AIDS in Africa focused almost entirely on efforts to prevent new HIV infections. This included behavioral education and condom promotion, HIV counseling and testing, treatment of sexually transmitted diseases (STDs) that can facilitate HIV transmission, and prevention of mother-to-child transmission. We tried everything we could to keep infections at bay.

And while preventing new infections is a critical part of any infectious disease response, HIV/AIDS quickly taught us that there are limits to what general prevention efforts can achieve in the absence of treatment or vaccines.

Why?

First, HIV/AIDS prevention was a mixture of measures that could mean nothing or everything: abstinence messages, disease information, condoms, and to some extent, testing. Diffusing this information and interventions to the whole population—many of which would never be infected in the first place—was expensive. Also, the virus remained an invisible threat unless you got hit by it or you saw a close relative hit by it. If you feel a threat from a rocket or a bomb, you can measure the impact.

How do you visualize a threat from a microscopic virus like HIV unless you watch its impact? Human nature is optimistic and built on hope. We never think it can happen to us, so why worry about preventing it? For example, campaigns against smoking lasted for years with little effect. It was only when advertising by cigarette manufacturers was banned and smoking was no longer allowed in public spaces that smoking prevalence dropped. Yet general prevention remains popular because it is easier to implement than targeted interventions. It can also, at times, be used by political leaders as an opportunity to exercise power over the whole population in the name of "protection." We seem to have forgotten the limitations of general prevention during COVID-19—instead of protecting the most vulnerable, we shut down entire countries and economies.

Second, prevention methods are influenced by social, structural, and environmental factors, including poverty, class disparities, structural racism, stigma, and gendered power differentials.

For example, in Rwanda, wearing a condom was often seen as an admittance of wrongdoing.

We often saw men denying the riskiness of their sexual behavior or denying any extramarital sexual relations that may have resulted in their positive diagnosis—often blaming their wives for their diagnosis. My friend, Joel, who ran two cohorts of pregnant women, often shared stories of HIV-positive women who were stigmatized by their communities and families and accused by their husbands of having given them HIV. Their husbands, meanwhile, would refuse to get tested themselves and would resist any intervention that would help prevent further transmission.

In our sex workers cohort, I saw several incidences when women were forced to have unprotected sex for fear of losing a customer. A few less customers meant the difference between eating and not eating that week. Celine, one of the women who came into our clinic, told me many of her clients refused to wear condoms. She said insisting they did would put her ability to provide food for her young son at risk. She knew exactly what needed to be done, but she had no choice but to take the risk to raise her child.

The challenges we faced with voluntary counseling and testing (VCT) are other good examples of the societal barriers to disease prevention. VCT is an HIV intervention that includes both voluntary pre- and post-test counseling and voluntary HIV testing. People, of their own free will, opt for VCT, and it provides them with an opportunity to confidentially explore and understand their HIV risks and to learn their HIV test results. When an HIV-positive person became aware that they were infected and received appropriate counseling, they were better able to cope with the disease and take action to protect their partners from infection. Similarly, people who knew that they were HIV-negative, especially in a high-prevalence area, found encouragement to reduce risky behaviors and protect their health. This is why voluntary counseling and testing programs were thought to be one of the most promising prevention tools we had at the time, and a key entry point for HIV/AIDS prevention, care, and support. At least, that was the idea.

But broad-based community participation in voluntary counseling and testing is often difficult to achieve. Discrimination against HIV-infected people discourages many from seeking testing and counseling services. Fears of stigmatization and the possibilities of domestic violence and desertion by husbands and family were also strong barriers to women joining.

While in Rwanda, my wife Marie-Helene, who is a nurse by training with a public health degree, worked at a VCT center called Centre d'information, de Documentation et de Councelling (CIDC). Marie-Helene told me stories of women who were the primary attendants of CIDC. Unlike Grace, who happened to not use a condom on one particular night, the women Marie-Helene served were forbidden to ever protect themselves by husbands who often came home drunk and aggressive and refused to put on condoms. In fact, the high-risk behavior was not coming from those who came to be tested, but from those who didn't. How do you deliver the messages then? Again, we felt helpless. And these are just a few of the many stories we heard every day in Rwanda.

Despite our best efforts to promote general prevention methods, we repeatedly ran into one roadblock—the absence of medical treatment for HIV/AIDS. Without access to medical treatment, patients had much to lose and little to gain by knowing their status. Why know that you have HIV if there is nothing you can do about it? There is a growing body of evidence suggesting that the availability of treatment advances prevention goals. In other words, prevention and treatment support each other.

The reason is one I've mentioned many times in this book already: there is more to medicine than science. Most of all, there is the human factor. Prevention solutions that disregard inherent human psychology and social practices—be it testing without treatment or locking down cities during COVID-19— don't work because humans are going to be humans. Most are not going to change the behaviors they've practiced their whole lives, in particular if doing so threatens their broader well-being. If they are going to change anything at all, it needs to be easy and practical. Does that mean we need to disregard prevention measures altogether? Not at all. But we need to strive for prevention measures that are simple for the average patient—a mask to protect from a respiratory disease is a more effective solution than an education program for the masses on why COVID-19 can kill you, for example. These prevention measures should complement a collaborative effort to develop and make treatment accessible as quickly as possible—or a vaccine, the most effective prevention method by far.

It was here that I had my first thought on access. I was in Rwanda to help set up cohorts that would make it possible to expedite HIV vaccine trials in hope of getting it to people as soon as possible. People enrolled in the cohorts received education and tools like condoms to prevent the disease. Those that did become sick received treatment for opportunistic infections. Those were two things that would not have been available to them outside the cohort. It was a positive step forward, but time was ticking, and people were dying all over Rwanda and Africa. As time passed, it became clear to me that once we found a vaccine, developing countries like Rwanda may not be the first to access it. And it wasn't just an issue of the cost of the vaccines. How could we reach patients in a country with such little healthcare infrastructure to actually get them vaccinated? That thought didn't leave me from that day forward, and it is still relevant thirty years later as developing countries struggle to access COVID-19 vaccination.

As the search for the HIV/AIDS vaccine continued, disease

incidence rose despite general prevention methods—not just in Rwanda, but everywhere. By the end of 1993, we reached the exponential phase of the epidemic. Cases were skyrocketing at an unprecedented pace. There were an estimated 13 million AIDS cases globally.

In the absence of an effective vaccine or treatment, we couldn't just give up. We had to find a better way.

Chapter 4

VIRUSES ARE SMART

The origin of the human immunodeficiency virus (HIV) has been the subject of scientific research and debate since the virus was identified in the 1980s. AIDS is caused by two types of retroviruses, which are viruses that affect the immune system. These are HIV-1 and HIV-2.

Using the earliest known sample of HIV, scientists have been able to create a "family-tree" ancestry of HIV transmission, allowing them to discover where HIV started. Their studies concluded that HIV originated from SIV (simian immunodeficiency virus), a related virus that attacks the immune system of monkeys and apes. It is believed that the first transmission of HIV took place around 1920 in Kinshasa in the Democratic Republic of Congo, likely as a result of chimps being killed and eaten, or their blood getting into the cuts or wounds of people while hunting. The earliest known case of infection with HIV-1 in a human was detected in a blood sample collected in 1959 from a man in Kinshasa. But as far as we know, the virus stayed put at that time. Why? It's hard to say for sure, but it mostly comes down to habitat.

When humans encroach on animal habitats, like forests for example, it creates opportunities for closer contact between animal species and humans. Eventually, viruses once found only in a specific animal species now have an entirely new category of hosts—the human. This is how H1N1 (bird flu) moved from birds to humans, how MERS did the same, and most recently, it is likely how COVID-19 transitioned from a disease found in a few people in Wuhan, China, to infecting millions all over the world. In 1959, monkeys still roamed free in their habitats with little human intrusion. This meant that while the virus could cross over to humans in isolated episodes, it didn't happen sufficiently for the human form of the virus to become the dominant strain. It also helped that a person in 1959 Kinshasa was not boarding the next flight to Europe, Asia, or the United States.

Unlike plants, animals, and other organisms, the only way a virus can reproduce is by entering a host cell, such as that of a human, bird, or monkey. It does so by attaching its surface proteins to the cell's membrane and entering the cell.

Once inside the cell, the virus instructs the host cell's machinery to make more viruses. The virus replicates thousands of times in a day, causing the host cell, which is now loaded with viruses, to explode. This, in turn, sends viruses in every direction, including into other cells, creating multiple infected cells. But host organisms are not passive observers to this process, and over time, a human's immune system can learn from these encounters and develop strategies to prevent reinfection. The next time the same virus comes to a host cell, it may find that it is no longer able to attach to the cell's surface membrane. So to survive, a virus must adapt or evolve, changing its surface proteins enough to trick the host cell into allowing it to attach. But how do they do it?

Every time a virus replicates, there is a chance the virus's genetic material (DNA or RNA) will mutate. With thousands of replications happening daily, some of the new viruses end up with a changed surface protein. If the host doesn't react to the dominant strain of the virus, nothing really happens. However, if the host starts reacting and killing the dominant strains, then this leaves a large opportunity for the mutants who have changed their surface proteins to bind to the host cell and replicate and become dominant. This is how new COVID-19 variants came to be. Mutant, or variant, strains become dominant when the prevalent strain becomes constrained by an unfavorable environment.

This is not only a characteristic of viruses. It is a common feature for all living species. In 1859, Charles Darwin published *On the Origin of Species* in which he outlined the principles of natural selection and survival of the fittest. Natural selection works by giving individuals, animals, or organisms who are better adapted to a given set of environmental conditions an advantage over those that are not as well adapted. For animals and humans, this process of evolution takes thousands and millions of years to materialize because the replication cycles are counted in months and years and the environmental constraints are slow-moving. For bacteria and viruses, the replication cycles take a fraction of a second, allowing mutations to emerge in a matter of days and weeks.

Viruses are smart. Their intelligence is genetic. They are living organisms, and like us, they are focused on survival. To keep their species alive, they need to reach as many hosts as possible, people included. The smartest viruses don't kill their hosts because that would prevent them from multiplying and spreading. Herpes hominis 1 is one of the smartest viruses. The Herpes DNA stays with you all your life and transmits to others episodically through "fever sores." HIV is similar, but slightly less smart because, in the end, it kills the host several years later. Ebola, on the other hand, is a significantly less intelligent virus because it kills 90 percent of infected people in three to five days after the onset of symptoms. It also is transmissible via body fluids when the subject is symptomatic—precisely when other humans would avoid making the contact necessary to facilitate transmission. This is why Ebola outbreaks are short and typically contained.

COVID-19 is smart too—many asymptomatic cases and relatively low death rates mean the virus can easily spread, mutate, and adapt. Under strict lockdowns, the virus had less room to replicate and spread. So it mutated into more contagious variants capable of spreading despite lockdowns and other restrictions as less contagious variants died off. The less contagious and usually more deadly variants of COVID-19 died off along with the person it infected. We see this pattern with many viruses, like the flu for example. The flu virus mutates regularly. That's why we are vaccinated annually against the flu. Every year, vaccine manufacturers make small changes to the vaccine so that it targets the most widely circulating virus.

Epidemics and pandemics aren't new. They have been a continuous threat to humanity and living animals since bacteria and viruses first appeared on our planet 4 billion years ago. In fact, microorganisms like bacteria, viruses, and fungi have been around for much longer than humans. These tiny organisms have adapted through major cataclysmic shifts, including (and most impressively) through all five major ice ages, when most other forms of life were wiped out. They managed to survive every time because of their incredible ability to adapt to their environment. We tend to forget just how resilient bacteria and viruses are—much more resilient than humans, in fact.

As long as we continue to think that we can overcome infectious diseases, we will remain vulnerable to preventable disasters, and as long as we think that we are powerful enough to overcome these microscopic organisms, we will remain unprepared to deal with them.

When it comes to viruses, we have to learn to live with them—in the same way they adapt to us.

It's something I didn't fully understand until I experienced the evolution of the HIV/AIDS pandemic.

HIV attacks immune cells called T helper cells that normally protect against invaders like HIV. If enough T cells get destroyed, it leaves your body defenseless against the virus and other "opportunistic" infections. Plus, HIV is with you for the long term. RNA viruses that cause a cold, a flu, and COVID-19 "visit" the host, stay a bit, and then leave after replicating and transmitting to other hosts. HIV, however, is a DNA virus. That means it blends into the DNA of our immune system and stays there for life by tricking your body's host cells to make multiple copies of it.

However, something both DNA and RNA viruses have in

common is their ability to mutate and change over time. That is why, like COVID-19, there are several different strains of HIV. HIV-1 tends to be more contagious and mutates frequently, creating several subtypes. HIV-2 is less contagious and evolves much more slowly.

In the early '90s, scientists began identifying different subtypes of HIV-1. By the mid-'90s, we had begun to see significant variation in HIV prevalence rates, or the proportion of people in a certain population who have a disease, across different parts of Africa. Within Sub-Saharan Africa, the AIDS epidemic was noticed first in Central Africa. Soon after, the epidemic was observed in East Africa, and subsequently in West Africa. The epidemic seemed to occur last in Southern Africa.

In Rwanda, as with other East African countries, HIV incidence was around 15 percent of the total population, with subtype B the most prevalent circulating strain. In West and Central Africa, a less infectious subtype A was the most prevalent, infecting an average of 5–6 percent of the population. Subtype C, however, which is found in Southern Africa, is known as a particularly infectious and contagious strain of HIV. Incidence in the region sits at 25–30 percent—the highest in the world.

As our knowledge of HIV evolved, we also made a significant finding: not everyone is susceptible to HIV/AIDS. Through our discordant couples cohort, run by a professor from the University of California, San Francisco, we saw a growing number of cases where one part of the couple was infected, but not the other. While tracking HIV in pregnant Rwandan women, she found that 14 percent of her 1,500 research subjects did not share the same HIV status as their partners. Before this study, scientists believed spouses would always share the same HIV status.

I remember one couple well—Benedict and her husband. She was negative and her husband was positive. It took many, many hours of convincing for the husband to agree to wear condoms. "If she didn't get infected before, why would she now?" he asked. I am not sure he was ever fully convinced. Maybe I remember because of my experience with Grace. In her case, one night of unprotected sex with her boyfriend changed her life forever. It was a stark contrast to Benedict's story. HIV was a cruel disease, and to this day, we don't know everything about why some people get infected but not others. In fact, we will never know everything about HIV, or any other viruses and bacteria. These microorganisms are unpredictable and much, much smarter genetically than us.

As the complexity of HIV/AIDS became increasingly evident, it triggered all of us working in public health to think about prevention and management in a more targeted way. In the beginning, we focused on general prevention. We didn't know who was going to get infected and wanted to prevent the disease in the greatest number of people. But we had already established, as I told you in the last chapter, that general prevention is neither efficient nor cost-effective. We couldn't continue to design general prevention interventions assuming that every country and everyone was equally susceptible to the disease. Instead, we had to target our interventions.

Around the same time, economists Mead Over and Martha Ainsworth, in the World Bank Policy Research Report titled *Confronting AIDS: Public Priorities in a Global Epidemic*, touted the medical and economic merits of targeted interventions—with a particular focus on those most likely to transmit the disease and those most vulnerable.[4]

The report essentially changed how HIV prevention was conducted. While we knew that the impact of prevention interventions was limited, in the absence of treatment, we shifted gears to targeted prevention mechanisms in hopes of better success.

In Rwanda, we began to target prevention interventions to those most vulnerable to being infected based on their behavior, and to those most likely to transmit the virus to others. Interventions were based on behavior because we didn't yet know why some were more medically vulnerable than others. For example, we began to put specific emphasis on empowering vulnerable populations to overcome societal barriers. We focused on positive, psychosocial support for sex workers, so they didn't feel stigmatized and rejected and instead felt empowered to act by proactively asking their clients to wear condoms. Many of these sex workers felt at the mercy of their clients who either refused to wear a condom or were too drunk to put one on.

Another example involved our previously mentioned voluntary counseling and testing (VCT) cohort, run by Colette at CIDC. To reach the most vulnerable with our VCT efforts, we needed to conduct education and communications in high-risk areas. To help us do that, Greg, Colette's husband, who was a professor of geography, mapped every bar and club across Kigali to help us target the type and timing of our interventions. We also fig-

---

4   Martha Ainsworth and Mead Over, Confronting AIDS: Public Priorities in a Global Epidemic, a World City Bank Research Report (New York: Oxford University Press, 1997).

ured out when most men in the region got paid for their jobs. Many would immediately visit bars upon getting paid, which eventually led them to sex workers—making it an ideal time to make sure the men and women had what they needed to prevent transmission.

These examples in Rwanda were only a small sliver of the targeted prevention work happening around the world at the time. It was only the beginning of what was to become a much bigger global movement for targeted prevention interventions. We hadn't figured it all out, but we had learned that a one-size-fits-all approach to prevention isn't effective and costs a fortune. When I first arrived in Rwanda, it was a blank slate. Now, slowly but surely, the pieces were starting to come together.

Before I tell you more about Rwanda, I think it's important to reflect on this important moment in the world's HIV/AIDS response. The shift to targeted interventions wasn't just a trend. It completely changed how public health practitioners viewed the effort, manpower, and funding required to respond to a public health threat, making us much more effective and, in turn, saving many lives. That is why it's so hard to understand why thirty years later, we seem to have forgotten it all. By the time COVID-19 hit us, the global HIV epidemic had long ago disappeared from the news, mostly seen as an issue for countries without the proper resources to manage it. Many public health officials seemed to be of the frame of mind that today's world was much better prepared to stop an outbreak and that global pandemics were a thing of the past. Our science had evolved, and so had our systems. Something like HIV couldn't happen again in this day and age. Or could it? It could, and it did.

I developed COVID-19 myself early in the pandemic. I can't confirm it, though, because there were no tests available yet. I think I picked it up on my way back from a business trip in Asia. I lost my sense of taste and smell and had a terrible fever. I felt awful. I couldn't move a muscle and spent much of my time in bed reading every bit of news I could find on COVID-19. I couldn't believe what I was reading. It was as if the world had never dealt with an infectious disease outbreak before.

By the end of February 2020, panic set in, and the world was reeling. After China, Italy was the next to shut down its borders and lock down its population on February 23, following a rapidly deteriorating outbreak. France soon did the same, and so did the rest of Europe, Asia, the United States, and Latin America. As an epidemiologist and as someone who had been at the frontlines of HIV, it seemed so obvious that shutting down would do more harm than good. We needed targeted prevention focused on protecting the most vulnerable, not locking up entire populations.

Yet in March 2020, Imperial College London offered one of the earliest projections of COVID-19 deaths around the world. It predicted 2.2 million fatalities in the United States and 510,000 deaths in the UK in the absence of control measures in just three months.[5] In reality, there were 385,000 deaths in the United States during the entirety of 2020. The model assumed all people are equally vulnerable to COVID-19, yet we know that this is not how viruses work. During the HIV/AIDS pandemic,

---

5 Neil M. Ferguson et al., *Report 9: Impact of Non-Pharmaceutical Interventions (NPIs) to Reduce COVID-19 Mortality and Healthcare Demand*, Imperial College London, March 16, 2020, https://doi.org/10.25561/77482.

similar models assumed entire villages and cities in Southern Africa would be wiped off the map. It didn't happen!

Different people react in different ways because everyone's immune system reacts differently to viral aggression. Although we don't know exactly why yet, we have many examples to prove that this is how viruses act. Despite this, Imperial's forecast became a guide for public policy and a key impetus for aggressive measures to control the virus's spread, including closures of businesses, schools, and places of worship, a pause on commercial activity, and travel bans. We've become so dogmatic in our approach to healthcare that we failed to apply the learnings of the past. We began the COVID-19 pandemic with a blank slate, as if we had never dealt with anything like this before. Yes, the virus was different, but the foundation was there. We just chose to ignore it.

As expected, the lockdowns did little to quell the virus. Governments grew desperate, eager to avoid more deaths and the public relations nightmare that follows a failing public health response. One by one, they made the decision to lock down their borders and shut down their economies. Everyone was to stay home.

But not quite everyone, right? Because we need people in our hospitals to take care of the sick. People to run our electricity grid to keep our houses powered. We need people to farm and produce the food that keeps us alive, work in the factories that prepare that food for consumption, and bring it to our stores. These people fall into the category of "essential workers." When you think about it, a significant part of our population is made up of essential workers. In France, for example, it's around 50 percent. So when governments told us to stay home, much of the population did not have the luxury to do so. These essential workers went to work, came back home, and infected their families and households. In lower-income countries where the essential worker context may be less relevant, the prevalence of multi-generational households, small living spaces, and the need to leave the home daily to collect food or go to work created similar problems. The world's double standards were on full display. That is why lockdown doesn't work in rich and poor countries and why cases plateaued but remained high and immediately shot back up once cities opened up again. Unless governments are able to keep every single person in their homes and guarantee that they are not interacting with anyone else outside their direct household, lockdowns have limited, short-term benefits and long-term consequences.

Consider this. On April 11, 2020, Imperial College London, the same group that had issued the earlier report that panicked governments, issued a study saying that in France, 2,500 deaths were prevented as a result of confinement—while at the same time, there were over 12,000 deaths.[6] That means that the death toll would have been 15,000 without lockdown—that's 16.6 percent efficacy. If this were a vaccine, would you take it knowing it could only protect you 16.6 percent? Did it make sense to shut down entire economies for a disease with an average global 1–2 percent case–fatality ratio (the number of deaths per the number of confirmed cases)—a rate that has been declining steadily since May 2020? I don't mean to be insensitive to the many lives lost to COVID-19. Every life is

---

6   Seth Flaxman et al., Report 13: Estimating the Number of Infections and the Impact of Non-Pharmaceutical Interventions on COVID-19 in 11 European Countries, Imperial College London, March 30, 2020, https://doi.org/10.25561/77731.

important, but public health is called that for a reason. It's about putting measures in place that will protect the greatest number of people. If we look at the socioeconomic consequences of locking down, it's hard to make a case that it was worth it. In fact, a *Nature* analysis published in December 2020 found that less disruptive and less costly interventions—like public education, social distancing, or limiting event sizes—can be as (and sometimes more) effective than drastic measures like a national lockdown.[7]

I could go on and on about the unnecessary magnitude of the socioeconomic impact of COVID-19. But it didn't have to be this way. We could have taken a more targeted approach that focused our efforts on those more vulnerable to COVID-19 and let those less likely to be severely impacted by the disease to continue their lives with proper precautions. Like we did in Rwanda with HIV/AIDS. It didn't take long for scientists to figure out who was most vulnerable to COVID-19—the elderly, those with weak immune systems or lung or heart conditions, as well as diabetic and obese patients. We had the knowledge to make the decision to target our prevention efforts. But we didn't have the collaborative geopolitical environment needed to mobilize a unified, science-driven response guided by past learnings. We also didn't have the mechanisms to easily iden- tify and isolate vulnerable patients because of our antiquated healthcare system. Many lives were lost as a result.

✶ ✶ ✶

7   Nina Haug et al., "Ranking the Effectiveness of Worldwide COVID-19 Government Interventions,"
     Nature Human Behaviour 4, no. 12 (December 2020): 1303–12, https://doi.org/10.1038/
     s41562-020-01009-0.

Less than a year after we arrived in Kigali, just as our cohorts were coming together and we were beginning to learn so much, the Rwandan Civil War reached a boiling point.

The Rwandan Civil War was fought between the Rwandan Armed Forces, representing the country's government, and the Tutsi rebel Rwandan Patriotic Front (RPF) from October 1, 1990, to July 18, 1994. The war arose from the long-running dispute between government-aligned Hutu and rebel Tutsi groups within Rwanda. In late 1993, there was hope for a peaceful settlement between the two ethnic groups. A small faction of RPF settled in the parliament in Kigali to allow more comprehensive and intensive talks. A transitional government with moderate Hutus was put in place. Everyone was looking forward to a peace deal.

On the evening of Wednesday, April 6, 1994, an aircraft carrying Rwandan president Juvénal Habyarimana and Burundian president Cyprien Ntaryamira, both Hutu, was shot down with surface-to-air missiles as it prepared to land in Kigali. Responsibility for the attack is disputed, with most theories proposing either the RPF or Hutus opposed to negotiation with the RPF.

Marie-Helene saw the plane being shot down from the terrace of our house that evening as I was putting my two boys to bed. The assassination set in motion the Rwandan genocide, one of the bloodiest events of the late twentieth century. Chaos ensued immediately.

Everything moved very quickly. The plane came down on a Wednesday evening. That night, we heard some gunshots followed by a morbid silence until dawn, when the Rwandan

Presidential Guards began killing moderate government members. Shooting soon commenced between the Rwandan Armed Forces and the RPF. By Thursday afternoon, there was rampant killing across the country. Tutsi homes were targeted systematically, people were killed, and bodies were loaded in trucks.

I drove our babysitter, Lillian, who happened to be Tutsi, home that Wednesday night as violence ensued. I remember discussing whether it was better to keep her with us, but she preferred to go home to her family given the circumstances. Lillian lived close to the parliament, where the shootings started early Thursday morning. Her area was among the first to be attacked. She was killed along with 30,000 Tutsis in those first few days. I often think about what could have been if she stayed with us instead. We knew right away we had to leave. We began packing up our things and on Friday morning, women and children, including my wife and two boys, were flown out on a French military plane headed to Bujumbura in Burundi. I was evacuated the next day to Bangui in the Central African Republic. For several tumultuous days, my wife and family didn't know where I was until we finally reunited in Paris. But of course, we were the lucky ones.

In the end, the Civil War resulted in 500,000 to 600,000 Tutsi deaths. A few years later, the conflict extended to the eastern part of then Zaire, now the Democratic Republic of Congo (DRC). People in the eastern part of the DRC have very little in common with those in its capital Kinshasa and west DRC. They are separated by 1,000 miles of equatorial forest. They were closer to people in Rwanda, Burundi, and Uganda. But the equatorial forest was rich in diamonds. This is why the colonial powers kept it in the same "country" during the Versailles Treaty in 1919. These borders were drawn the way they were to keep the diamonds all under one country, under their control. The situation in Rwanda and Zaire only strengthened my belief in the danger of antiquated borders and systems put in place by our ancestors and deemed untouchable to enable control and cover up human intolerance. Much like in Lebanon as a kid, where I saw my life crumble before my eyes because of tensions between Shias, Sunis, and Christians.

After Rwanda, I started seeing the world differently, looking across borders, searching for commonalities and ways to overcome the many unnecessary divisions holding our society back, including our healthcare system. I didn't know what it was yet, but I knew we needed a better solution.

Chapter 5

BIRTH OF UNAIDS

Despite all that happened in Rwanda, Africa taught me what it meant to live freely, and this feeling didn't fade over the years. It is difficult to explain why. Maybe it's because Africa's "modernization" didn't happen to the extent that we see on other continents. Think about it—countries are often organized into two categories—developed and developing. But what is actually developed or developing in these countries? It's their systems and structures to support and protect their populations. These systems bring order, which is generally thought of as a good thing. But the order tends to breed rigidity. The rigidity that envelops our daily lives in more developed countries only became clear to me when I visited a part of the world where it was not nearly as present. Does it have to be that way? I'd argue that it's not necessary for rigidity to accompany progress. There is a way to build a system that thrives on common values and not a generalized mistrust that must be controlled by a growing list of laws and regulations. That learning guided the next chapter in my life.

Soon after returning to Geneva in the summer of 1994, we learned that an HIV vaccine would not work any time soon. Traditional vaccines, like the measles, mumps, and rubella (MMR) vaccine and the pneumococcal vaccine, are often made by using weakened or inactive versions of that virus. These weakened or inactive versions of the virus prompt your body to create antibodies that tell the virus that you've already been infected, causing it to die off. But HIV wasn't deterred by antibodies. It lived in our DNA instead. Once in the body, HIV stays with us forever. We don't recognize it as a foreign body, and so we can't use a vaccine to fight it. Other viruses like herpes and Epstein-Barr do the same, but HIV is the deadliest. To this day, science hasn't found a way to target DNA viruses.

The news dealt me quite a blow. Despite the work that had gone into it, I felt like we had created hope among communities in Rwanda. And that hope was now gone. I had to find another way to help.

Back at WHO, I met with a Dutch professor who was a leading scientist in the search for an HIV treatment and was running WHO's Care and Treatment Department. He asked if I wanted to transition to the group working on Prevention of Mother-to-Child Transmission of HIV/AIDS, known as PMTCT. It was a hot topic in the world of HIV/AIDS with some promising research on the horizon. I was eager to get involved and was honored to work with him. He was a visionary. I have no doubt his work would have continued to save many lives today, but sadly, on the way to the AIDS Conference in Malaysia in 2014, he was one of the AIDS researchers who died on the Malaysian Airlines flight shot down over Ukraine.

Under my new role in the PMTCT group, I would be taking the spot of a doctor I coincidentally had worked together with at Claude Bernard hospital in Paris and have been close with ever since. When I went to Rwanda, he took over my desk at WHO, and when I came back to Geneva, I took over his job when he was given a new assignment in Ethiopia as project manager for the Ethio-Netherlands AIDS Research Project (ENARP). Global health is a small world, as you can see. Many of the same people do everything. It is quite insular, which, despite how brilliant these scientists are, contributes to the rigidity of the health system.

It was a good opportunity to apply what I had learned from the Rwandan cohorts. The mid-'90s were a turning point for HIV/ AIDS, and I had no intention of stepping away. Incidence continued to rise and targeted prevention was taking center stage. But it was becoming increasingly evident that it wasn't enough. We needed to do more, and we needed to do it quickly. We felt it, and the WHO member countries told us the same. In the 1990s, thirty-six new countries joined WHO, more than any other decade—a reflection of the global optimism and spirit of collaboration of the post–Cold War era. Now, these countries were demanding more.

As I've already told you, HIV was not only a medical problem. Given the fact that the disease lasted a lifetime, it induced stigma, social inequalities, and economic burden. It also broke apart families and communities. If we were to make a dent in a disease that was then infecting more than 20 million people around the world, a coordinated, multisectoral response would be needed. One that prioritized not just targeted prevention but the availability and accessibility of treatment. Without treatment, prevention efforts would only go so far.

WHO's donor countries identified the need for a joint program on HIV/AIDS to help expedite our global response, forming in 1996 what is known today as the Joint United Nations Programme on HIV and AIDS (UNAIDS). Led by Peter Piot, UNAIDS was to be "the main advocate for accelerated, comprehensive and coordinated global action on the HIV/AIDS pandemic."[8] UNAIDS initially brought together six United Nations system co-sponsors—UNICEF, WHO, UNDP, World Bank, UNFPA, and UNHCR—to enable the type of multisectoral response the HIV/AIDS crisis required. That kind of multisectoral, collaborative response could have been very helpful during COVID-19. UNAIDS was and still is today the only co-sponsored joint program in the United Nations system. With political will behind it, UNAIDS went on to become a key driver and player in the unified global response to HIV/AIDS. Under my new role focused on Prevention of Mother-to-Child Transmission, I became part of the UNAIDS response.

The birth of UNAIDS came at a time when cross-sector and cross-regional collaboration and optimism reigned supreme. The "New World Order" was starting to materialize not just on the healthcare stage, but in the political and economic world as well.

One example took place in South Africa, beginning in 1990 with the release of Nelson Mandela after twenty-seven years in prison. Following the historic moment, the government of Pres-

---

8   "UNAIDS Profile," OAS, updated June 11, 2013, http://www.oas.org/en/ser/dia/institutional_relations/ Documents/Profiles/UNAIDS.pdf.

ident F. W. de Klerk began repealing much of the legislation that provided the basis for apartheid—the archaic system of segregationist policies against the country's non-white citizens since 1948. A new constitution giving new rights to Black citizens and other racial groups took effect in 1994, and elections that year led to a coalition government with a non-white majority. This coalition did what for decades seemed impossible—it brought an end to the hateful apartheid system.

Around the same time in the northern hemisphere, the United States, Britain, and countless other global partners came together to liberate Kuwait from Iraq during the Gulf War. A few years later, in 1995, NATO and its partners helped end the gruesome Balkan War. These three events had one unifying takeaway: the use of collaboration to solve large problems. It's a defining characteristic of the "New World Order," and hence, the spirit of the time.

In fact, in the same year NATO intervened in the Balkans, the World Trade Organization (WTO)—an intergovernmental organization that regulates and facilitates international trade between nations—also commenced operations. Its purpose was to facilitate trade in goods, services, and intellectual property among participating countries by providing a framework for negotiating trade agreements and reducing potential trade barriers. The WTO would go on to be the world's largest international economic organization, with 164 member states representing over 96 percent of global trade and global gross domestic product (GDP).

In becoming members of the WTO, countries commit to eighteen specific requirements, including the Trade-Related Aspects of Intellectual Property Rights (TRIPS). TRIPS introduced intellectual property rules into the multilateral trading system for the first time. It facilitated trade in knowledge and creativity and helped resolve trade disputes over intellectual property, while ensuring WTO members were still able to achieve their domestic objectives. In the coming years, the TRIPS agreement would have a significant impact on the pharmaceutical sector and access to medicines.

The geopolitical context of the mid-'90s was one ripe for collaboration and progress. As a product of its time, UNAIDS capitalized on this spirit to form a global movement against HIV/AIDS.

For those of you not around at that time, the best way I can describe it is to compare it to the honeymoon stage of any new relationship. Everything seemed possible. We had plenty of ideas, and governments desperate for solutions to the growing crisis were willing to listen. Every door was open for us. Borders suddenly became less important when it came to the HIV/AIDS response.

I remember hearing about a company that made female condoms, called The Female Health Company. Women are about four times more vulnerable than men to sexually transmitted diseases, including HIV. This is largely because of anatomy: the area of the female genitals exposed to semen and other sexual fluids during sex is four times larger than that of men. The cells forming the mucosa of the vagina are less resistant than the skin covering the male genitals. Women are also at more risk of getting infected because semen contains greater amounts of the virus than vaginal fluids. As part of our growing concentration on targeted interventions, WHO decided to do a study on female condoms to assess their effectiveness in preventing transmission and feasibility of use. The study's target population was sex workers in Thailand—one group would use male condoms and another group would be given the choice to use a male or female condom. There were many issues associated with male condoms—some of which I observed firsthand in Rwanda. Sometimes condoms weren't available and sometimes they would break. Some partners of sex workers—whether they were the husband or a client—refused to wear a condom, and some were too drunk to put one on. We were hopeful that female condoms could be a method of giving women more control over their own health. The study ultimately found that when women had the choice of both a male and female condom, they had significantly less unprotected sex and got one-third fewer STDs than those given only the male condom.

Once we knew that it could be a feasible solution, we went to the company to inquire about mass manufacturing and how to make it available worldwide. I traveled with Brian, a business consultant hired by UNAIDS who had long experience working with pharmaceutical and healthcare companies. As soon as we got to the offices of The Female Health Company, Brian looked around and told me: "Not much is happening in this company…" I asked later how he guessed. He told me that usually, you find papers on the tables, boxes ready to be sent, couriers waiting on the secretaries' desks. Here everything was too clean. As the meeting progressed and after signing a confidentiality agreement, it quickly became clear that they were on the verge of bankruptcy.

Yet all of us at UNAIDS agreed that we had a responsibility to increase awareness of this public good. But the price of female condoms in low- and middle-income countries was between US $2 and $3. This was much too high for the populations who are most likely to benefit from it. To make female condoms more affordable, UNAIDS negotiated a discounted rate with The Female Health Company, dropping the price below US $1. In an unconventional move, and without any interest other than the provision of a public good, we became pseudo marketing managers overnight. We reached out to all the Ministries of Health to share our study results and put them in touch with the manufacturers. Orders started coming in—enough to keep the company afloat and to provide an alternative to particularly high-risk groups.

We also partnered with Population Services International (PSI). I knew them from Rwanda, where they were doing a remarkable job. PSI utilized a method where a product was made commercially available at a fraction of its actual cost, and the remaining cost was subsidized by governments and donor organizations. The method uses typical marketing practices to promote the product and build demand, but unlike traditional marketing, the end goal is not profit. It's called "social marketing." It was just what we needed. I called PSI's vice president and asked if they could take on the project. UNAIDS could initiate the demand but didn't have the capacity to sustain the work. Knowing him, I knew he wasn't the guy to back away from a challenge. He told me that launching an entirely new product—especially such an unconventional one for the time—would be very difficult, but he also agreed that it was not the time for a conservative attitude. We reached an agreement and PSI took over the management of the orders and marketing until The Female Health Company got back on its feet.

Unfortunately, while still available today, female condoms never achieved the same level of popularity as their male counterparts. Some say it's because they were noisy. Others blame a lack of public education and promotion. Others see it as a de-prioritization of women's health. I think it's a little bit of all those things. But the fact that in 1995 we managed to get traction on a solution that remains taboo more than twenty-five years later says a lot about the spirit of borderless collaboration, openness, and flexibility of the time.

Chapter 6

TREATMENT CHANGES EVERYTHING

We haven't talked much about medications to prevent HIV/ AIDS or to treat existing patients. That's because for nearly a decade from when the virus began wreaking havoc on the world, there were few available options. In low- and middle-income countries, options were even more limited.

The first turning point came in 1987, when researchers discovered that a failed cancer drug from the 1960s, zidovudine (ZDV), also called azidothymidine (AZT), stopped HIV from multiplying and helped people with AIDS live slightly longer. It became the first HIV medication available to the public. Early AZTs unfortunately did not cure the disease or prevent opportunistic infections altogether, and they couldn't prolong a patient's life for more than a few months at best. They also had significant side effects. But the lack of alternatives for treating HIV/AIDS at that time meant patients had no choice but to deal with the unpleasant side effects, and physicians had no choice but to prescribe a medication they knew would cause their patients to suffer. Despite these limitations, these early generation drugs, which belonged to a drug class called nucleoside reverse transcriptase inhibitors (NRTIs), were hugely significant because they showed that treating HIV was possible.

In the early 1990s, additional NRTI drugs gained FDA approval. They were able to extend a patient's life by a few months, but they also had their drawbacks. They didn't sufficiently reduce the impact of the virus and also came with some nasty side effects. At the time, AZT was also the most expensive prescription drug in history, with a one-year price tag of around US $3,600 (equivalent to US $6,840 in today's dollars)—clearly beyond reach for much of the world.

It also didn't work so well on its own. Pascal was on AZT alone and it didn't save him. HIV replicates swiftly and is prone to errors each time it does. These errors, or mutations, cause small changes in the virus that can result in resistance to a regimen. Remember, viruses are smart and are preprogrammed to keep their species alive—just like humans. In some people taking AZT alone, drug resistance developed in a matter of days. For that reason, scientists began to test whether combining drugs would make it difficult for the virus to become resistant to all the drugs simultaneously.

During the early '90s, several different combination therapies were studied and found effective.

While the effects of two-NRTI therapy were better than those of single-drug therapy for many people with HIV, they weren't always long-lasting. A major advance came in 1996 when researchers found that triple-drug therapy could suppress HIV replication to minimal levels. By preventing the HIV virus from replicating, and hence mutating, triple-drug therapy, also called highly active antiretroviral therapy, or HAART, also prevented drug resistance. These drugs cost, on average, US $12,000 per year back then, prohibitively expensive for most.

The possibility and success of HAART was partially due to the appearance of a new antiretroviral drug class—the protease inhibitors. In December 1995, saquinavir became the first protease inhibitor to receive FDA approval. With HAART, many patients saw the amount of HIV in their blood drop to undetectable levels. But while HAART was lifesaving, it was still far from perfect. The side effects were burdensome, and the daily dosing was complex. Certain drugs had to be taken in combination at different intervals throughout the day, some with food and some without. The complexity made it difficult for people to adhere to the regimens long-term. But we now had a light at the end of the tunnel. Protease inhibitors showed that AIDS no longer had to be a deadly disease. It was a hugely significant scientific accomplishment that shifted the paradigm of how the world saw AIDS and AIDS treatment. Overnight, despite high costs, public demand for saquinavir grew exponentially.

A year later came yet another class of antiretrovirals, called non-nucleoside reverse transcriptase inhibitors (NNRTIs). They were cheaper and easier to produce than protease inhibitors and they didn't require refrigeration, which was a major hurdle in low-income countries where the majority of HIV patients lived. Clinical studies had also begun to identify different effective combinations of NNRTIs and AZTs that simplified dosing regimens.

Thanks to these factors, the availability of NNRTIs became a major turning point for treatment access in resource-limited settings. But it didn't come easy.

In 1996, the ACTG 076 study showed that a regimen of zidovudine, or ZDV, one of the early treatments that I mentioned at the start of this chapter, provided to pregnant HIV-positive women starting between week fourteen and week twenty-eight of pregnancy until delivery and to the baby for six weeks, reduced HIV transmission to the child by two-thirds. A typical pregnancy cycle in humans is thirty-nine weeks. This implies fifteen to twenty-four weeks of treatment. In rich developed countries, this is possible because women are followed closely from the time their pregnancy is confirmed, which typically happens between six and twelve weeks. In low- and middle-income countries where healthcare facilities are not available everywhere, women would typically visit a facility no earlier than at thirty-six weeks. Many would just come for their delivery or choose to deliver at home. It was clear to the research community that the treatment regimen used in the trial would not be feasible in low-income country settings where mother-to-child transmission rates were highest. To make it work, we had to find shorter regimens.

A global effort began to test the effectiveness of less intensive, shorter treatment regimens with a greater potential for scale-up in those settings. With 1,600 babies born every day with HIV, most of them in the developing world, we needed this treatment as soon as possible. Under my new position as the coordinator of PMTCT research at UNAIDS, I was tasked with establishing an international working group to harmonize PMTCT studies from around the world.

By this point, it was clear to me that if we asked research agencies across the world to join in their official capacity in a formal international working group, we would be bogged down in political, diplomatic, and bureaucratic deliberations and spend months putting the group in place. There was no time for that. We were in the middle of a public health emergency and needed to work fast. I suggested that we set up an "informal" working group where experts leading PMTCT groups at their respective agencies would join the group in an informal capacity, making it not legally binding. Any research group or agency doing a trial on PMTCT was welcome to join the group. We met quarterly, which created personal bonds over time and broke the competitive barriers that are common among researchers. Free of formal approvals and bureaucratic constraints, this group was able to act quickly, harmonize study designs, and adapt its approaches. It turned out to be extremely effective. It is certainly a model that I went on to repeat many times later in my career.

We proactively decided as a group on questions we wanted to answer before research started and developed harmonized guidelines, methodologies, and protocols that would enable researchers from around the world to compile and compare their individual study findings. In total, there were twenty studies, each evaluating different combinations of medicines. While the research questions varied for each study, they complemented each other in a way that enabled us to answer many potential research questions on PMTCT at the same time.

The United States, including the National Institute of Health (NIH) and the Centers for Disease Control and Prevention (CDC), as well as French and Belgian academics, joined the informal group, along with Thai, Australian, and Canadian researchers. It was truly a global initiative. The informal nature of the group allowed leaders from major research agencies to participate in their personal capacity. At first, some resisted the informal nature of the group, but eventually, they came on board when they saw that several prominent researchers had already joined our effort. Over time, free from the usual bureaucracies, it became more powerful, and certainly more efficient, than a formal group.

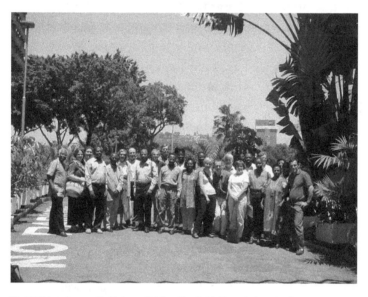

The PETRA study team I led in front of Mulago Hospital in Kampala, Uganda. This group included researchers from around the world working to find a combination of therapy that would be feasible in lower-income settings to help prevent transmission of HIV/AIDS from mother to child.

Eventually, a series of clinical trials of short-course ZDV began around the world to help find a simpler regimen for PMTCT. In all, sixteen trials were launched in low- and middle-income countries, including the Ivory Coast, Uganda, Tanzania, Malawi, Ethiopia, Burkina Faso, Zimbabwe, Kenya, Thailand, the

Dominican Republic, and South Africa. Nine of the studies were funded by the US CDC and NIH; five were funded by other governments, including Sweden, France, and South Africa; and the one I was running was funded by UNAIDS.

These trials had been cleared by ethics boards, yet they were labeled unethical by the advocacy community because researchers did not provide ZDV to all participants. Instead, in fifteen of the studies, women received placebo pills despite the fact that ZDV had already been shown to help prevent mother-to-child transmission of HIV/AIDS. Although research ethics protocols typically state that placebos should not be used when proven treatments already exist, in this case, the proven treatment regimens would have been completely infeasible for women in low- and middle-income countries. This was our rationale for including placebos in many of our trials. The purpose of our trials was to compare the already proven complex regimen to a simpler regimen. What if we found, after conducting the trial, that the simpler regimen was not as effective in preventing mother-to-child transmission? What would be the point of showing that a regimen not feasible in a country works better than one that does? Instead, we wanted to show that a simpler regimen was sufficient to achieve the desired outcome and better than nothing at all for women who cannot take the more complex regimen.

In 1997, the US activist group Public Citizen issued a letter to Health Secretary Donna Shalala. Here's a brief excerpt:

> Unless you act now, as many as 1,002 newborn infants in Africa, Asia and the Caribbean will die from unnecessary HIV infections they will contract from their HIV-infected mothers in nine uneth-

ical research experiments funded by your Department through either the National Institutes of Health (NIH) or the Centers for Disease Control and Prevention (CDC). Even though an NIH-funded randomized, controlled trial (so-called Protocol 076) demonstrated in 1994 that the antiviral drug AZT (zidovudine) can reduce transmission from mother-to-infant by approximately two-thirds, a finding so dramatic that the study was stopped prior to its scheduled completion, some or all of the women in these nine developing country experiments are still not being provided with effective prophylaxis, placing their infants at risk for fatal HIV infection. Instead, they are offered either placebos or interventions that have not been proved effective. In addition, 502 infants in six similar experiments funded by foreign governments (France–two studies, Belgium, Sweden, and South Africa) and the United Nations AIDS program will contract HIV, making a total of 1,504 infants who can be expected to die unnecessarily in these experiments, some of which are already underway. The dangerous double standard being practiced here is underscored by the fact that both U.S.-funded studies being conducted in this country provide AZT or other known effective anti-HIV drugs to all women, while only one of the 16 studies in the developing world provides AZT to all study groups. Providing AZT prophylaxis to pregnant, HIV-infected women in research studies in developing countries is clearly feasible; six developing country studies other than the one mentioned above provide AZT to some (but not all) of the women in the studies. In each of these six studies, one group of women is given a placebo instead of AZT. In essence, the U.S.-funded researchers are conducting experiments abroad that would never pass ethical muster in the U.S.[9]

---

9   Peter Lurie et al., A Letter to Secretary Donna Shalala, April 22, 1997, https://www.citizen.org/wp-content/uploads/1415.pdf.

On September 18, 1997, an editorial appeared in the *New England Journal of Medicine* denouncing the conduct of clinical trials in Africa, Asia, and the Caribbean that were designed to determine the efficacy of interventions to reduce maternal–fetal transmission of HIV.[10] The attack, signed by Marcia Angell, MD, the *Journal's* executive editor, further escalated the issue. That same year, Dr. Angell wrote the following in a *Wall Street Journal* op-ed:

> All the rationalizations boil down to asserting that the end justifies the means, which it no more does in Africa than it did in Alabama. It is easy to see the findings of the Tuskegee study from a safe distance of 25 years. But those so offended by the comparison of the African research with Tuskegee have yet to show how these studies differ in their fundamental failure to protect the welfare of human subjects.[11]

Conducted between 1932 and 1972 by the United States Public Health Service and the CDC, the Tuskegee Study was conducted with nearly 400 African Americans with syphilis to observe the effects of the disease when untreated. However, by the end of the study, treatment was available. Participants were never told of their diagnosis and treatment was never made available to them despite its availability. More than one hundred died as a result.

As the person coordinating many of the research groups mentioned in this letter, I can tell you firsthand that we spent

---

10   Marcia Angell, "The Ethics of Clinical Research in the Third World," *New England Journal of Medicine* 337, no. 12 (September 18, 1997): 847–49, https://doi.org/10.1056/nejm199709183371209.

11   Marcia Angell, "Tuskegee Revisited," *Wall Street Journal*, October 28, 1997, https://www.wsj.com/articles/SB877990421541676000.

days discussing each of these ethical issues. The trials were designed to compare the experimental, shorter regimens against a placebo, on the grounds that this reflected the current standard of care in these countries. This was the reality. Most of the researchers in our PMTCT group lived in Africa and low-income countries at some point in their life, and like me, they understood the double standards that exist between poorer and wealthier countries well. We of course wish that women in Africa had all the same luxuries as pregnant women in the US or Europe. Yet the reality was that they didn't, and trying to apply some idealistic goal to find a solution that wouldn't work in the African context wasn't going to help anyone. It's an ethical dilemma, I know. But in this case, an "equitable" solution would have been an ineffective one.

In a formal public response to the article in the *New England Journal of Medicine*, David Satcher, then director of the CDC, and Harold Varmus, then director of the NIH, stated that only placebo-controlled trials could provide "definitive," "clear," "firm" answers about which interventions worked in lower-income settings to help governments make "sound judgments about the appropriateness and financial feasibility of providing the intervention." Satcher and Varmus argued that comparing a simpler regimen of unknown benefit against the proven, more complex regimen, which is likely to be more effective, would be of little use if the more complex regimen would not be feasible for patients. They also pointed out that without a placebo control, it would be difficult to clearly determine whether the less complex but potentially less effective intervention is better than no intervention at all. Finally, they emphasized that the design of these placebo-controlled research studies had been built in consultation with country scientists and physicians.[12] We didn't design these trials while sitting comfortably in our offices in the US and Europe. We all worked closely with our counterparts in the countries where these trials were to happen. We traveled extensively to the locations to understand first-hand how it could work. We visited maternity wards, talked to women, and spoke with the midwives, nurses, and doctors before we designed the trials. Satcher and Varmus concluded that placebos were necessary to help policymakers make costly treatment access decisions in the face of scarce public health resources.

But activists are activists. Satcher and Varmus's argument was not enough for them. They continued to bash the agencies and the researchers. As the coordinator of the international working group on PMTCT, I had to step in and argue in support of the use of placebos. Some told me that I needed to remain neutral as a UN official and not interfere. By doing that, however, I would be betraying the members of my group, all of which had agreed on a clear way forward. Most importantly, I would have been betraying what I knew was right. This was not me. I decided to step into the battle encouraged and helped by the then UNAIDS Director of Communications and the head of the public relations agency working for UNAIDS.

During the day, I did countless interviews with European, Asian, and African media to try to educate and better explain the issue. Every night after putting my three boys to bed in Geneva (Paul was the last addition after we left Rwanda), I talked to US

12 Harold Varmus and David Satcher, "Ethical Complexities of Conducting Research in Developing Countries," *New England Journal of Medicine* 337, no. 14 (October 2, 1997): 1103–5, https://doi.org/10.1056/nejm199710023371411.

media. This wasn't a fair period for my wife, but she was always encouraging me because she believed it was the right thing to do. Others, like a prominent South African pediatrician who struggled during the apartheid and who was also leading a trial on PMTCT, stepped in as well. His voice was important as it was coming from the same countries the activists purported to protect.

This saga lasted for a year, until the results of the trials started to become clear.

For example, one of the working group's studies I was closely involved with, HIVNET 012, found that a single 200 mg oral tablet of a lower-cost ARV called nevirapine taken by the mother at the onset of labor and a single, smaller oral dose of nevirapine to be given to the newborn within seventy-two hours of birth significantly reduced the risk of HIV transmission. One pill of nevirapine reduced the transmission by 50 percent as compared to six weeks of daily treatment reducing it by 67 percent.[13] This was a game changer. It meant that one pill given to the mother and one single dose given to the baby made it 50 percent less likely that that mother would transmit HIV to the baby. Is 67 percent better than 50 percent? Yes, of course, but it's a moot point, because six weeks of treatment wasn't feasible in these environments. Patients would have to come back to a clinic to receive their medication multiple times—a clinic that could have taken them several days to reach by foot. They would also need to seek out treatment far earlier than was the norm in

13   Laura A. Guay et al., "Intrapartum and Neonatal Single-Dose Nevirapine Compared with Zidovudine for Prevention of Mother-to-Child Transmission of HIV-1 in Kampala, Uganda: HIVNET 012 Randomised Trial," *The Lancet* 354, no. 9181 (September 4, 1999): 795–802, https://doi.org/10.1016/S0140-6736(99)80008-7.

many lower-income countries—often only at delivery. Instead, this new nevirapine regimen could be given to the woman and the baby right at delivery, and it was more affordable too.

When the HIVNET 012 study results were made public, they quickly became the subject of an international media frenzy. I presented the results of the study to a crowded room at the retrovirus meeting in Washington, DC, and in what seemed like a few minutes, the news was everywhere. I sat in a room and took media interview after media interview. Overnight, we went from foes to heroes and the placebo controversy quickly took a back seat.

In 1998, one of the working group studies, which looked at 393 pregnant women in Thailand, found that women who took AZT during the last four weeks of pregnancy and during labor were 51 percent less likely to transmit HIV to their child than those receiving placebo pills.[14] The course cost a tenth of the standard treatment. Once the Thailand results were announced, we stopped using placebo controls. The placebo controls were important to prove how effective the shorter treatment regimens could be, but after the strong data from the HIVNET 012 study, followed by the results in Thailand, it could no longer be justified.

In the end, the conflict came down to an idealistic versus a pragmatic and incrementalist vision of the world. This mentality was prevailing in public health, and while it was intended to create equality, it further cemented the double standards

---

14   Nathan Shaffer et al., "Short-Course Zidovudine for Perinatal HIV-1 Transmission in Bangkok, Thailand: A Randomised Controlled Trial," *The Lancet* 353, no. 9155 (March 6, 1999): 773–80, https://doi. org/10.1016/S0140-6736(98)10411-7.

between rich and poor patients. Ideally, we all want to ensure that all women get the same level of care. But this idealism would have led to more inequalities because women in Africa wouldn't have gotten PMTCT interventions at all. There are not enough resources in the world to enable everyone to receive the same. Plus, the world is different. What works here doesn't necessarily work there. The only way to give everyone the same thing is to give everyone the lowest. Is that a better solution?

Let's look at an example outside of healthcare to help explain this issue. Take the iPhone. Imagine if, when Steve Jobs introduced the first iPhone, we asked for it to be available everywhere and to everybody at the same standard. But many people in the world don't have access to the internet, can't afford to pay even a fraction of the phone's cost, or have little use for the luxuries made possible through a smartphone. While the iPhone may have completely revolutionized the lives of those in richer countries, for many in the world, an iPhone has no use. It's nothing more than a rectangular pile of parts. Does that mean we shouldn't make it available to anyone? In my opinion, no. Waiting for the ideal only slows us down. We need to start with what we have and make improvements as we go. One may say that the iPhone is not the same as a medicine that is badly needed. This is true, but new medicines are also new technologies. They are tested, improved, streamlined, and distributed on a large scale. Constricting our research in the ACTG 076 box would have failed these HIV-positive pregnant women in low-income countries and would have left them to their fate.

Once all the studies from the working group were published, we decided as a group to conduct a meta-analysis to compare and contrast results and build upon each other's findings. To do so, we all had to share our data. Which all of us did, without pause. This level of data sharing and transparency was unprecedented then, and still is today, driven by competition among research groups and academia. All the trials conducted by the study group participants covered different scenarios and used comparable methodologies so we could compare results across trials. These weren't "me too" trials to assess whether your drug is better than mine. Before any trials started, we came together and figured out all the different scenarios and conditions we needed to test to get to a solution fastest. And that's exactly what we did. The meta-analysis showed that all the ARVs studied worked to significantly decrease the chance of transmission from mother to child. That was powerful because it proved that we now had a host of solutions in our hands for pregnant women and their babies.

The progress we made in no more than two years for PMTCT is undoubtedly a direct result of the collaborative, hopeful, and innovative spirit of the time—driven by the changing forces of globalization and a few individuals who chose to stand up to the status quo and do things a little differently. The entire scientific community was speaking in one voice, one message, and one set of recommendations. Science was making the decisions. If we had buckled under the pressure and didn't move forward with the placebo studies, we would have likely had to accept results that weren't practical for low- and middle-income country settings. I am so glad we didn't.

This kind of collaboration of the scientific community would have been invaluable during the COVID-19 pandemic. If today we could have done what we did with the informal working group, with countries and researchers working together, we could have saved so many lives, made vaccines available even quicker, and distributed them uniformly across the world. Instead, the change in the geopolitical climate, and divided policymakers and scientists too scared to go against the grain in fear of the constant pressure from often unvalidated opinions broadcast on social media, made it impossible. And more than six million people died as a result.

In the end, I am thankful to the activists whose passion pushed the issue to new heights and us scientists and researchers to new levels of collaboration. The placebo controversy brought global attention to the issue of HIV/AIDS treatment. There are not too many examples in history when so much of the scientific community joined together for one cause, making a deliberate decision to align our voice for the greater good. Although dealing with the criticism and questioning was frustrating, it also pushed us forward and ultimately toward identifying evidence that would completely change the paradigm for HIV/AIDS treatment in low- and middle-income countries.

The early days of HIV/AIDS treatment were messy and turbulent. But through it all, we can't forget to recognize the game-changer that was treatment availability. With treatment, we no longer had to shoot in the dark. Once treatments became available, public health engines shifted from reactivity to proactivity. Treatments create hope, and with hope comes faster, better science, more timely decisions from policymakers, and of course, more engaged patients who now have a reason to believe in better. Treatment changes everything. It allows us, physicians, health workers, public health experts, and policymakers, to change the course of the disease. Now that it was there, we had to find a way to make it widely available.

Chapter 7

A CHICKEN AND EGG SITUATION

The development of new HIV/AIDS regimens for pregnant women in low- and middle-income countries drew so much international attention that once they became available, the media temporarily stopped covering the HIV/AIDS situation in these countries. It was like the issue was solved.

But in reality, it was just beginning.

In fact, while activists and scientists debated how clinical trials should or should not be conducted, a bitter irony remained. Triple-therapy had become the standard of care in rich countries. It turned HIV/AIDS from a death sentence to a chronic disease requiring lifelong treatment, yet poorer countries were living a different reality. Even at significantly discounted costs, most of these countries couldn't afford these treatments for their population. For example, a treatment regimen for a pregnant woman then cost around US $800, a price affordable only in industrialized nations where PMTCT represented a limited problem. In Uganda, for example, that cost represented 400 times the then yearly per capita expenditure on healthcare. Nor did they have a healthcare system able to deliver them systematically to patients. How do we get these medicines to the people who need them? The availability of treatment and actual access to treatment are two very different things.

Most researchers feel that this should be someone else's problem. Their job is to do the research. Getting it to the patient is someone else's responsibility. This makes perfect sense, but it wasn't what I felt. I wanted to finish the job.

As the scientific community was following these discoveries, we at UNAIDS started wondering how we were going to deal with these major treatment innovations. UNAIDS had a mandate to lead the world when it came to HIV. It put together an internal task force to discuss what it would take to make treatment accessible worldwide. Being in the Care and Treatment unit, I was part of it. There were many aspects to consider: health provider education, availability of treatment guidelines, laboratory capacity to diagnose and monitor treatment, and supply chain infrastructure.

But the elephant in the room was the cost of treatment. Who is going to pay for these millions of people? Can we get pharmaceutical companies to lower their prices for low-income countries? After all, what is the point of having an innovation if the majority of people can't benefit from it? While this isn't a new question, HIV brought it to the public consciousness. Driven by a now more globalized world, all of us, from

Europe to the US to China to Africa, became keenly aware of the growing double standards that permeated every aspect of society—with healthcare, these double standards were bound to have significant repercussions.

We were asked who among the task force would be interested in engaging pharmaceutical companies. None of us had real pharmaceutical experience, including me, and most were hesitant to align themselves in any way to the big bad wolf, or any private company for that matter. I wasn't sure what to expect, but I was curious to find out what was possible. After all, the high cost of specialty medications didn't seem like an issue that was going away any time soon. We had to address it head on. I decided to raise my hand, and without much competition, was given the assignment. Brian, who had worked with me on the female condom project and had more experience working with pharmaceutical companies, was hired as a consultant to work with me on the initiative. He was excited by the challenge and so was I. We were determined to make it happen.

* * *

In 1997, pharmaceutical companies mostly followed one pricing model—one size fits all. The idea of pricing medications differently for different people was an unknown concept. It opened the door to a philosophical debate: should a product be priced according to its intrinsic value or what someone can pay for it?

When you go to your corner supermarket, you are paying a set price for a product. That price is based on what is assumed to be the perceived value that the product provides to the consumer. A candy bar that you are going to eat in two minutes is cheap.

It may satisfy your appetite for the short term, but the value it provides to you, the consumer, is limited. A fair amount of money was invested by the manufacturer of the candy bar to find just the right chocolate and the perfect combination of sweet ingredients that the greatest number of people would like, but it still doesn't compare to the millions spent by pharmaceutical companies to develop and test a new medication.

When I was in Rwanda, I found out that Jacques, my Rwandan counterpart, bought meat and vegetables at significantly cheaper prices than me. I initially felt annoyed and fooled. Jacques told me that they will never sell me the food at the market at the same price as his. "Why?" I asked Jacques. "My tomato is no better than yours." Jacques smiled and said, "These people at the market grew the tomato. They didn't attribute a particular value to it even if it has one. They know that you can pay more than I. They will ask you to pay more and they will find it unfair that you pay the same price."

A pill that can prevent you from dying from HIV/AIDS is clearly of high value to the patient using it. But what if most people who need this treatment can't afford it? Shouldn't we start thinking like Jacques?

With Brian, we began by visiting pharmaceutical companies one by one and asking what seemed like simple questions: Are you willing to lower your list price for countries unable to afford it? What does it take to make these products accessible to people in low-income countries?

At first, many companies told us it wasn't their problem. The companies' mandates were to discover and make the medicine.

They felt it was the responsibility of governments to give it to their people. The pharmaceutical industry in the '90s was different than it is today. Companies were largely developing primary care and infectious disease medications, which are cheaper to manufacture and are sold in huge volumes, making them more affordable. However, low- and middle-income countries had very little access to specialized medicines for more complex diseases primarily because their cost made them inaccessible to both governments and the general population. Unlike primary care or infectious disease medications, specialty medicines were much more difficult and time consuming to manufacture and were typically for conditions that affected a smaller group of people. High research costs and low volume contributed to their high cost. The truth is that this was the first time pharmaceutical companies were asked to compromise on price. It's also true that at this time, low- and middle-income countries were just simply not on their radar. Most countries were buying generic products with expired patents. There were also no patent laws in place to protect intellectual property, which meant companies had little financial incentive to invest in these regions. New medications often start off as branded products sold by pharmaceutical companies until patents on those products run out, enabling many generic manufacturers to create their own, often cheaper versions.

The pharmaceutical industry was also concerned about what would happen in their primary markets if they reduced their price in lower-income countries. If antiretrovirals, which I'll refer to as ARVs from now on, were made available in Africa and Asia at a lower price, how could they ensure that it wouldn't be resold in Europe or the US at a lower price? Would the governments in rich countries force them to lower their prices to the level of Africa and Asia? Who can give assurances that this is not going to happen? And if companies were to lower their prices, did we have evidence that these countries had the infrastructure to deliver these drugs to patients properly and securely? It was a fair question. At the time, the answer was no.

When we spoke to governments in developing countries, they had their own hesitations. They asked why they should invest in building up their infrastructure for products they cannot afford without company commitments to lower their prices. It was another fair question.

It was a chicken and egg situation.

Meanwhile, activist groups in the United States and Europe were working hard to bring the public's attention to the issue of treatment access and expedite a solution. Groups like ACT-UP, Public Citizen, AIDES, and Médecins Sans Frontières were focused on a single solution to the pricing crisis: generics.

Activist groups had no interest in working with pharmaceutical companies to negotiate price reductions mostly because they didn't believe that companies would ever stick to a reduced price. Instead, many wanted companies to open their patents to generic manufacturers via compulsory licensing. Compulsory licensing refers to when a government allows someone else to produce a patented product or process without the consent of the patent owner or plans to use the patent-protected invention itself. The patent owner still has rights over the patent, including a right to be paid compensation for copies of the products made under the compulsory license. They believed that by creating competition, prices would go down—instead, it prevented pharmaceutical manufacturers from competing at all.

The World Trade Organization (WTO) had just commenced operations with more than 164 member countries. In becoming members of the WTO, as I mentioned earlier, countries agreed to adhere to several agreements, including the Trade-Related Aspects of Intellectual Property Rights. TRIPS, as it's more commonly known, introduced a minimum global standard for protecting and enforcing intellectual property rights, including those for pharmaceutical patents. TRIPS also gives countries a certain amount of freedom to modify regulations to enable a proper balance between the goal of providing incentives for future inventions of new drugs and the goal of affordable access to existing medicines. Compulsory licensing is one of those flexibilities. While TRIPS doesn't provide a list of acceptable reasons to justify compulsory licensing, it does provide several conditions for issuing compulsory licenses, such as a public health emergency. It also states that the person or company applying for a license has to have tried, within a reasonable period of time, to negotiate a voluntary license with the patent holder on reasonable commercial terms.

Yet many activists, staunchly against the pharmaceutical indus-try, saw generics via compulsory licensing as the only solution. In my opinion, it was another idealistic solution that wouldn't solve the problem in the long term. The public health com-munity has always had a tendency to push one-size-fits-all solutions for a very diverse world. Protease inhibitors were difficult to make, and we knew it would take years for generic manufacturers to be able to replicate them. To this day, generic manufacturers have not developed generic protease inhibitors.

But even if I didn't fully agree with them, activists played a very important role. Their tactics made it impossible to look away. When one pharmaceutical company declared a 50 percent reduction in their price, I remember activists staging a sit-in in front of the home of an executive of a competing pharmaceutical company with leaflets marked with the word "assassin" in hopes of getting them to do the same. It garnered international attention and pushed pharmaceutical companies in ways they had never been pushed before. US and European activists also helped activism gain traction, for the first time, throughout Africa and in other low- and middle-income countries. Hearing directly from people in the countries most affected was powerful.

The media also put pressure on pharmaceutical companies and governments. Most of the media coverage focused on the major gaps in access to treatment in developing countries, but few talked about how to solve the problem—until I met Mike Waldholz, a prominent health reporter at *The Wall Street Journal*. He had previously covered PMTCT issues and was fascinated by the idea of using different prices in different settings, as he wrote in the foreword of this book. He felt it was needed and unprecedented. Michael helped us indirectly by bringing public attention to the idea in well-balanced articles that presented both sides of the issue and didn't bash it from the start.

But still, we saw little movement. We were at a standstill. No one was willing to budge, and meanwhile, people were dying by the millions every year. Whose responsibility was it to solve this issue?

In August 1996, in a well-read, highly publicized paper by Philip Musgrove titled *Public and Private Roles in Health*, the World Bank explored the idea of healthcare as a public good and opened the doors to the discussion around whose responsibility it was to solve the access to treatment issue:

Public goods are goods or services such that one person's consumption does not reduce the amount available for others to consume. Typically these are goods from which consumers cannot be excluded: if they are made available to anyone, they are available to all, at least locally or temporarily. Since people can consume such goods without having to pay for them, no one will produce them for sale to individual consumers. Therefore they will be produced only if government (or some other source such as a charitable organization) pays for their production. The notion of a public good is no different in health than in any other sector: wherever such goods or services are to be available, they must be financed by government or some other non-market alternative. […] the boundary between public and private goods is not sharply defined, because some interventions provide substantial externalities. In these cases, individuals can and do buy an intervention and benefit from it, but they cannot prevent non-consumers from also deriving some benefit. Because the purchasers do not capture all the benefit, they may be unwilling to pay for all of it: in consequence, private markets can exist but will produce less of these interventions than would be optimal for society as a whole. This problem arises most readily with communicable diseases, because the infected person puts others at risk. Curing one case therefore also prevents others. Tuberculosis control is a clear example: no victim of tuberculosis is likely to ignore the disease, so there is no problem of people undervaluing the private benefits of treatment. Rather, the cost of treatment—and the fact that they may feel better even though the disease has not been cured—may lead people to abandon treatment prematurely, with bad consequences not only for themselves but for others. The rest of society therefore has an interest in treating those with tuberculosis, and assuming at least part of the cost. Asymptomatic communicable diseases, such as some sexually transmitted infections, also create externalities; but because people may not realize they are infected, the demand for care is too low even when care is free (zero price). There is then an argument not only for subsidizing treatment, but for persuading those infected to seek care.[15]

In a nutshell, the statement declared that treatments for communicable diseases (or infectious diseases, as you may know them best) are a public good, assigning governments the responsibility of providing these treatments for their population. That's great in theory, but is it realistic? To provide treatment for their population, they must be able to pay for them. To pay for them, prices need to be within their means.

We were back at step one. To get unstuck, we needed to help companies and governments find common ground by actually showing and not just talking about potential solutions. Once again, we came back to that incrementalist pragmatic thinking that helped us navigate the placebo trials. We needed a proof of concept to demonstrate that access to treatment via differential pricing was possible. We had to show companies the commercial and social value of such an investment and that countries could manage to properly deliver these drugs to patients. This would reassure the companies that they were not embarking on a major transformation before knowing where they were going. It would also show governments that companies were in fact serious about their commitments. We needed to generate

15   Philip Musgrove, "Public and Private Roles in Health: Theory and Financing Patterns," *Health, Nutrition and Population Discussion Papers* (Washington, DC: The World Bank, 1996), https://documents1. worldbank.org/curated/en/357021468739572306/pdf/multiopage.pdf.

momentum with a solution that was tangible and concrete, not another discussion in a gray conference room.

By this point, my public health career had shown me many times that the perfect solution takes a long time to build. We couldn't let perfect become the enemy of good. We had to start small with a few countries and as many companies as we could get to follow. Once we proved the concept, the rest would come. Learn, adapt, build, and scale. That's exactly the sentiment that brought about the Drug Access Initiative.

Chapter 8

NEGOTIATING WITH THE BIG BAD WOLF

Nothing like it had ever been done before.

I discussed the concept of conducting pilot programs to assess the feasibility of ARV access in low- and middle-income countries with my boss at the time and with UNAIDS's executive director. They agreed that we couldn't continue to have hypothetical discussions with governments and companies that went nowhere. We had to put forward tangible options.

In November 1997, we decided to give the pilot programs a try, under what we called the Drug Access Initiative, or DAI. But where would we conduct them? We knew we wanted to represent different regions of the world in the countries we selected. We also had other criteria: the nations needed to be of manageable size to make the pilot possible and underdeveloped enough to serve as an example, and most importantly, they needed to have the political will to collaborate.

During our search, we cast a wide net and talked to countries around the world. Each had its own unique challenges. In Latin America, Brazil wanted to do its own thing. Argentina was in the Organisation for Economic Co-operation and Development (OECD) and its economy and infrastructure were too developed for this project. Many others were too small to show the scale we needed. We landed on Chile.

In Asia, the obvious choice would have been Thailand, but they were in the midst of a serious battle with pharmaceutical companies. Thailand was playing a leading role in the TRIPS negotiations and pushing for removing patents. Vietnam, on the other hand, was just starting to open up, and their government showed interest in such a program. Vietnam it was.

And finally, Africa. Uganda was the most proactive in Eastern Africa. Their Minister of Health had been pushing for greater access to treatment for some time already. On the west coast, in francophone Africa, we looked into Senegal and Côte d'Ivoire, and ultimately landed on Côte d'Ivoire because it was hit harder by HIV.

Now, we just had to get the pharmaceutical companies on board. This was easier said than done, of course. In order to have a decent triple therapy to offer patients, which was necessary in order to suppress the virus sufficiently, we needed at least three companies to agree to lower their prices.

Meeting after meeting, we heard the same thing from the companies we spoke with:

"We are not allowed to discuss prices between companies."

"This is contrary to antitrust laws."

"We need an antitrust lawyer in the room."

"Our responsibility is to discover and make the product available."

We expected it to be a bumpy road, and indeed it was. I found myself at the center of a major war on drug prices and pricing strategies.

Triple-drug therapy made price negotiations with companies close to impossible. Each pill was manufactured by a different company with different price expectations. Try getting three companies to agree on anything, let alone a common price. And the antitrust laws didn't help either. In much of the US and Europe, antitrust laws were in place to prevent companies from colluding on prices or even discussing pricing. We had to have an antitrust lawyer in the meetings or we needed to discuss individually with the companies. I've never been a fan of formal meetings—most don't achieve much. That's why we focused on individual discussions and kept formal meetings with antitrust lawyers to the bare minimum.

Over the span of three months, Brian and I met with every manufacturer of HIV/AIDS treatments more times than I can remember. We were an unlikely duo. I was the science and technical guy, and he was the commercial guy. He understood the pharmaceutical industry well and had great contacts. I knew what it took to get it done on the ground. We didn't always see eye to eye, and our approach in talking to companies wasn't always aligned. He felt I was doing too much listening. I thought he was doing too much selling. But looking back, we accomplished a lot together.

It started with Abbott, Bristol-Myers Squibb (BMS), GSK (then Glaxo-Wellcome), Hoffman-La Roche, and Merck. We knew that if we could get the major ARV manufacturers on board, the rest would follow.

Thankfully, we found one early adopter—GSK's then HIV franchise president. GSK was an important player in HIV and the most prominent manufacturer of ARVs. He knew well that access to medicines was not an issue that was going away any time soon. HIV/AIDS had opened the world's eyes to the double standards of healthcare and there was no turning back. He also felt strongly that companies had an ethical responsibility and an ultimate interest to ensure their drugs were not priced out of the reach of those who need the treatments most. The risk of having drug prices questioned in richer countries was not an acceptable reason to not lower prices in low- and middle-income countries. His early support not only helped bring GSK on board to DAI but also mobilized other companies to follow suit.

BMS wasn't as interested. Or at least not at first. I remember them telling us that they felt their role was to make medicine available, but the rest was the government's responsibility. They were also convinced that changing the price in Africa would prompt the US and EU to do the same—significantly deflating their major revenue sources.

Merck thought much of the same. They felt that if something

was to be done, it should be philanthropic, which was exactly what I wanted to avoid. We at UNAIDS were looking at long-term sustainable solutions and not short-term, feel-good philanthropic actions for media buzz.

Roche wanted guarantees. "How do we know products won't be bought at a lower price and sold for profit in more developed markets? If patients don't take the medicine and HIV cases in the country continue to rise, will people start to say our product doesn't work? Can the infrastructure in these countries handle storing and distributing these products?" We couldn't provide guarantees. All we could do was use DAI to put in place a system to avoid issues like product diversion. After a few more meetings, we were able to get them on board.

We had a tentative yes from two out of five, but how could we pin down the others?

Having BMS, for example, would have made a huge difference as they had didanosine, which made triple-combination therapy more effective. We pushed them by saying that by not participating, they would be turning their back on the bulk of their patients. It was hard to argue against that. Eventually, I could see that they had begun to come around. Some of their senior leaders had started to personally connect with the cause. It's one thing to push back when you are speaking as a company. At a human-to-human level, it's a very different thing to ignore the plight of millions of people. Once we had their buy-in, they played a significant role in convincing BMS's top management to sign off on their participation in DAI.

We also tried to get all the companies together for a collaborative meeting, but they refused to come without an antitrust lawyer. They worried they would be blamed for colluding to lower prices. We ended up with a "diplomatic" meeting where few spoke their mind, the discussions didn't address the real issues and concerns, and no conclusion was reached.

In the end, it was the dinner after the meeting that made all the difference. GSK's HIV franchise president, who I told you had been a strong proponent of DAI from the start, invited the group to a delicious meal of raclette (a strong-smelling but delicious Swiss meal famous in the region). We talked as humans, and had a frank conversation about the importance and weight of this decision to participate or not and what it would mean for patients. We stayed away from price discussions and focused on the benefits of the approach. By the end, we had all the companies on board. GSK, BMS, and Hoffmann-La Roche were the first to officially sign up. Abbott and Merck soon followed, along with Dupont, Organon Teknika, and Virco. At first, each company agreed to offer their medications at a 50 percent discount to countries participating in the DAI pilots. Later, that would go down even further to a 70 percent discount. Since then, I've concluded all my major negotiations over a nice meal.

A few weeks later, we were able to get an endorsement from the International Federation of Pharmaceutical Manufacturers & Associations, opening the door for other pharmaceutical partners. But we weren't out of the woods yet. Soon we were contacted by PhRMA, the Pharmaceutical Research and Manufacturers of America, furious that we were about to implement a major differential pricing program including American companies without involving them. Their concern—as you can probably guess—was that this would affect US prices. They weren't happy. There was nothing new about their argument. "This is highly risky," they said. "You haven't done this before." "If you had our experience, you wouldn't." "We've done something similar in the past, and it didn't work." I remember the discussion being rather condescending. The world was opening up, and here were these representatives from an industry that was supposed to be driving innovation, refusing to see past the status quo. It was extremely frustrating, but in the end, while having their buy-in would have been a strong bargaining chip for us, they didn't have the power to stop us, so we charged on.

Next, we moved to governments. Back then, the US and France were the countries investing the most in research.

We met with the US Surgeon General and the director of the AIDS office at the White House. A few months back, the US Surgeon General had pulled me aside during the World Health Assembly to say thank you for our efforts during the PMTCT trials. I told him about DAI and he expressed his support. When we met with him this second time, it was clear that he didn't want to implicate himself or the US government directly in what was likely to become a controversial topic. The director of the AIDS office at the White House expressed a similar sentiment, but both reassured us that they would not get in our way.

In France, our initiative was met with frank enthusiasm at the highest levels. French President Jacques Chirac even announced the establishment of the Fonds de Solidarité Thérapeutique International (FSTI), or French Solidarity Fund, to help several African countries access ARVs. There were many francophone countries in Africa that had been hit very hard by HIV and the French government was eager to show what they were doing to improve the situation. DAI came just at the right time. French support was a clear boost to our initiative right from the beginning. I'm eternally grateful to two close friends who were then part of the French Government and were instrumental in helping this Lebanese French doctor navigate French politics. The funds first went to the Côte d'Ivoire pilot, and over time the DAI model was used in other countries by the French government. The contribution was the first time there was public government support for ARVs and showed that there were, in fact, wealthier countries willing to invest money in this issue.

During all of this, I was working with a key lawyer at the World Health Organization to draft up agreements for the companies who would participate in DAI. She had a reputation for being tough. She was feared by many at WHO. She was extremely competent and detail-oriented. If you had to work with her on an agreement, you knew you had to have your ducks in a row. I still remember her face when I told her I needed agreements between four governments and five pharmaceutical companies done in a few weeks. "Are you crazy?" she said. Agreements of this kind took months, sometimes years in the UN. We weren't an organization known for speed. I invited her for lunch to discuss the details. The lunch took close to three hours and was followed by several others and many reviews. I passed by her office practically every day to check how things were moving along, and there were often questions, ideas, or thoughts to discuss. She saw the urgency and helped me get approvals in two months. That's ten minutes in WHO time. It was an incredible feat, and I credit her as one of the major drivers that made DAI possible. What we were trying to do was unconventional, and she could have easily stood behind the wall of bureaucracy and put an end to it. But she knew what was at stake. I am still so proud today of the small group of us at UNAIDS who managed to push through DAI knowing we were doing the right thing.

We had most of the parts in motion, but before we could really start, we couldn't ignore the activists. Some moderate organizations like AIDES and Treatment Action Group had started to come around and see DAI as a step in the right direction. But others, and particularly ActUp, the major US activist organization at the time, were still hung up on the idea of opening patents to enable generics and wanted nothing to do with any other solutions. They wanted access for all and saw these small pilots in select countries as unsatisfactory. They also saw them as a way for pharmaceutical companies to minimize their involvement in low- and middle-income countries and to build arguments against voluntary licensing. But relying only on generics would take years because generic manufacturers don't invest in innovation and in opening new markets. They come when the market is there. There was still no market in low- and middle-income countries. Where there is no money, there is no movement. We needed to open the markets first.

My communications counsel set up a meeting for me with ActUp. I thought there would be eight to ten people at the meeting at most. When I arrived, the meeting was in an amphitheater with one hundred people from ActUp and their allies. This was one of the most difficult meetings I have ever had. I had to find neutral ground we could all agree on, even if I didn't have 100 percent of their buy-in. If they turned against UNAIDS and the story got out to the media, all the pharma partners we had worked so hard to get would have backed out. They asked for guarantees of universal access. They asked for immediate access to generics and for patents to be dropped. I couldn't offer any of those things. Instead, I said, "I understand your arguments and your fight. Don't change it. With DAI, we can start treating patients in low- and middle-income countries in a few weeks. If you have a faster way to provide access, tell me now. If not, support us with this initiative while you continue your longer-time fight." I am not sure all of them were convinced. The UN wasn't known for getting things done. But at a time when everyone was looking for solutions, UNAIDS, via the PMTCT work and now DAI, was moving things forward. I think that helped give groups like ActUp some confidence. Eventually, they backed up and gave us the space we needed to move forward with DAI.

By this point, AIDS had become the leading killer in Africa. In Sub-Saharan Africa, HIV had infected 34 million people and killed 11.5 million since 1981, dwarfing malaria and tuberculosis. In 1998 alone, AIDS accounted for 1.8 million deaths in Sub-Saharan Africa, nearly double the 1 million deaths from malaria and about nine times the 209,000 deaths from tuberculosis.

Speed was paramount in this situation. With DAI, we had companies willing to offer a solution now for patients. Despite its start in only select countries, I saw that as a much better option than many more months of negotiations while patients continued to die. The intention was for DAI to become a model for access to treatment in the future. HIV was complex. It required viral load assessments, long-term follow-up, and psychological support for patients. There was no model for this kind of intervention in low- and middle-income countries back then, and we needed one urgently.

While everything wasn't perfect, we had to move. I remember Uganda's then Minister of Health telling me he couldn't hold his breath until the entire world agreed that equitable access was necessary. He needed solutions for his people now. Uganda became the first country to begin a pilot program.

Chapter 9

BRINGING TREATMENT TO AFRICA: THE STORY OF THE DRUG ACCESS INITIATIVE

With several companies on board and willing to offer their products for a discounted price through the Drug Access Initiative (DAI), we set out to take these pilots from paper to practice. DAI needed to demonstrate that with the proper approach, it was possible to overcome the challenges of drug access in the developing world and to do so in a way that was sustainable and replicable.

We needed to show that ARVs could be effectively sold, distributed, and used consistently by patients in low- and middle-income countries so that these pilots could be scaled nationally and across other countries as well. Will drugs reach patients and not be diverted? Will patients take and stay on their treatment? The regimen for protease inhibitors, for example, included more than fifteen pills a day. That's a lot to ask of a patient. Some treatments also had significant side effects. How feasible are these price reductions? How can we make these solutions sustainable so that countries could continue to build upon them for many years to come? Those were the questions we were trying to answer.

Answering these questions involved more than purchasing and distributing drugs, although that in and of itself was a tremendous financial and logistical challenge. We had to start by building a basic medical infrastructure in the pilot countries that would facilitate drug access and ultimately attract drug companies to the country in the future. That infrastructure included treatment guidelines, lab facilities, a referral system, healthcare worker training, an effective supply chain, patient education and follow-up mechanisms, and of course, a well-functioning regulatory and finance system to handle drug registration and money flow. It was a lot, and although we realized that no single program could solve all those challenges, we had to start somewhere.

Making sure that DAI could evolve into a longer term solution after the close of the pilot was important to us. To make that happen, we had to design the DAI pilots in a way that made it advantageous for all parties involved. We did this in three ways.

First, and I'd say most importantly, we created a model that we hoped would be economically sustainable. Patients would have to pay for their medication—but at a significantly discounted price. As I mentioned, at first, each company agreed to offer their medications at a 50 percent discount to countries participating in the pilot. They later lowered that further to a 70 percent discount. Paying for treatment helped ensure that patients saw the value of the medication they were receiving and were, in turn, more likely to take it as prescribed and to stay on treatment. It would also help ensure that companies didn't lose money so they had a vested interest in providing these medications for the long term.

Even with a 50–70 percent discount, there was only a small percentage of the population that could afford these medications. It wasn't the best scenario. I knew, and all of us working on DAI knew, but like I said, we had to start somewhere. Some access was better than no access. Plus, creating a marketplace for these drugs was a key part of our sustainability strategy. It was this marketplace, combined with an assurance that drugs could be distributed effectively, that would push companies to continue selling to these countries far beyond the end of the pilot and encourage other funders to come on board to further subsidize the cost for patients. In return, governments would also have more incentive to build the infrastructure needed to provide better care. In some countries, like Côte d'Ivoire, other partners came on board quickly. The French Solidarity Fund covered the cost of treatment for patients who couldn't afford it, so the medication was ultimately free to them.

Second, we put in place foundational pieces that would make it easier for countries to implement interventions like this in the future. For example, we worked with countries to establish a National HIV Drug Policy, coordinated by a National Advisory Board made up of local government and NGO representatives, medical experts, and a representative of UNAIDS. We also worked closely with the government to develop treatment guidelines. There were no ARVs in the country then, so doctors, pharmacists, and nurses had no experience dealing with them.

Third, we made sure supply chain systems were as reliable as possible and able to prevent product diversion. Our intention from the start was to improve the systems that were already in the country. But in many of the pilot countries, there was little to no infrastructure there to accept, store, and deliver high-cost, lower-volume drugs. Public supply chains were used to managing large bulk orders of generic medications—like aspirin. They didn't have the experience or infrastructure to manage smaller quantities of specialized, high-cost medicines and ensure a continuous supply of those medicines so patients wouldn't develop HIV resistance (a risk if ARVs are not taken consistently). Trying to adjust these systems to the needs of HIV/AIDS medications could have taken years and significant money—both of which we didn't have. Unfortunately, in some countries, building a system for drug delivery separate from the national system was necessary.

Uganda was one of those countries. Their Central Medical Stores (CMS) run by the government didn't have the capacity to sell products and had little experience storing and distributing expensive medications, which require more oversight to prevent product loss and diversion. Before we started, I remember meeting with one of the local World Bank representatives to check out a CMS warehouse that was reported to have just received a shipment of 200 big boxes of medicine to treat opportunistic infections in AIDS patients. I wanted to understand how the shipment was handled upon arrival—how it was processed, stored, and delivered to local health clinics and eventually to patients. The warehouse manager gave an impressive presentation of their processes, but when you looked around, you could see that there were only a few boxes in the warehouse. When I inquired about what happened to the shipment of 200 boxes, the manager didn't know. No one knew. They may have been distributed to the health center already, but the fact that nobody knew posed a clear problem of traceability.

The other major distributor in Uganda was called the Joint Medical Stores, which was a joint venture between Uganda Catholic Medical Bureau (UCMB) and Uganda Protestant Medical Bureau (UPMB). JMS was able to sell products, but they only handled large, bulk shipments. We need facilities to handle small quantities of high-value products.

Despite our intentions to use DAI to build up the country's existing distribution channels, like CMS and JMS, instead of creating new ones, without the luxury of time and money we had to build a parallel channel. To get ARVs into the country, we set up a nonprofit organization called Medical Access Uganda Limited that we set up with the Ministry of Health's approval to purchase the drugs from participating companies at a subsidized rate, then stored and distributed them to patients.

In Uganda, we hired a local pharmacist with a recently completed MBA, Sowedi, to run the operations, which he still runs today. Sowedi had an incredible entrepreneurial spirit and unmatched drive. From a one-room office on the second floor of a medical warehouse, he managed a two-person operation, negotiated with companies, managed importation and distribution, and kept track of every prescription and every patient who used medicines purchased via DAI. No one was doing that at the time. Medications were delivered to clinics and there was no feedback system to trace what was used, by whom, or what was stolen or thrown out. It was more about making sure stock was available, and not that the patient was actually taking it. For us, this was a major gap. As part of DAI, we made it a priority to link stock information with patient consumption and make sure medicines were getting to the right patients. How can we fight an epidemic if we don't know that patients are taking the medicine that we are working so hard to get into their hands?

To achieve this, we pre-qualified clinics that wanted to receive medications based on their ability and willingness to track drugs and patient consumption. We didn't care if they were public, private, missionary, or NGO entities. Public health tends to divide everything by public versus private, but there's no real benefit to doing so. We believed it was about capacity, not sector. Working with these clinics and pharmacies, we also set up mechanisms to track patients and make sure they were taking and staying on their medicine. This involved training pharmacists and health workers on the importance of keeping medical records, having clear stock cards that link stock data to patient data, and following up with patients to make sure they were taking their medications. There was nothing fancy about these processes, but putting them in place made a huge difference because it created a system that linked consumption to people to track treatment adherence, better estimate stock needs, and prevent stock diversion. The availability of patient-level data helped us achieve one of the major goals of DAI: to show clear evidence to pharmaceutical companies that ARV access in developing countries was in fact possible.

During these early days in Uganda, not everyone was open to

DAI. Many public health leaders thought the country's limited resources could be better spent on other critical health issues, like clean water, nutrition, or HIV prevention education versus treating a small number of HIV/AIDS patients. I also remember one instance with the Ugandan military. They sat us down and tried to intimidate us into providing the military with ARVs before the public. That kind of strong-arming was prevalent among these groups back then, and we were suggesting a different way.

Thankfully, we had a lot of support from the then Minister of Health. He knew he couldn't pay for treatment for all his people and was open to the idea of creating a market for ARVs to help kickstart access in his country. I remember meeting with him right before we launched DAI. He asked many questions, as usual, and truth be told, not everything was as buttoned up as I would've liked. The minister wasn't happy about it and questioned whether we should delay the launch. I was nervous to pull the trigger, but I knew that we couldn't wait for perfect. We just had to start. It was different than what he was used to, but with some trepidation, the minister agreed to take the risk with us. He gave us the freedom to try it a different way, knowing the current way wasn't working. A few days later, DAI started. His leadership is a key reason why Uganda was one of the first African countries to receive ARVs.

We were creating something completely new and facing immense local and international pressure to deliver—the world was watching. From that one-room office, Sowedi kickstarted a new reality for ARV access in Uganda. In a May 2000 *Wall Street Journal* article, reporter Mike Waldholz wrote:

What the UNAIDS program provides, at least in Kampala, is "reliability in access and price," says Sowedi Muyingo, who was hired by UNAIDS to be the general manager of the nonprofit company, Medical Access Ltd. "Even though the prices here are still too high for most people, the doctors who treat HIV patients know when they prescribe the drugs that we have a steady and secure supply at prices they can count on." Indeed, the U.N. is using the Uganda project as an example of what can be done in Africa when the government, foreign-aid organizations, and drug makers cooperate on a grass-roots level.[16]

DAI was ultimately about creating a model for access to ARVs that governments, companies, funders, and others could then replicate and scale to address the HIV/AIDS pandemic on a global scale. In Uganda, I learned that the model would need to be driven not just by better systems, but by dedicated people willing to push it forward. The Drug Access Initiative in Uganda was able to provide treatment to more than 1,000 patients and build the capacity of more than 146 health centers across the country at a time nothing else was available to them. Importantly, it also helped create a stable foundation for access initiatives to come.

In Chile, it was a different situation. The infrastructure was already there, and DAI ran in both the public and private healthcare systems; the latter supported 30 percent of the population. The supply chain infrastructure worked well. The most significant barrier we faced was a bureaucratic one with their VAT (value-added tax) system. All Latin American countries had World Bank and IMF loans, and as a result, all had put in place a VAT system to support the repayment of those loans.

---

16 Michael Waldholz, "Five AIDS Drug Makers Agree to Slash Prices for Poor Nations," *Wall Street Journal*, May 12, 2000, https://www.wsj.com/articles/SB958071884605755937.

What that meant was that import duties would be added to the cost of the drug, which had already been discounted by 50 percent. Clearly, it made little sense to add more costs to the patients via VAT when our main objective was to reduce the costs of treatment. Eventually, the Ministry of Health was able to provide a waiver specifically for ARVs, which finally made it possible for ARVs to enter the country under favorable terms for the companies importing them at a discounted rate. Private insurance companies also began including ARVs in their plans, making it possible for some patients to receive partial reimbursement. Over time, ARVs became fully reimbursed in Chile thanks to the progress kickstarted by DAI.

In Côte d'Ivoire, the Ministry of Health was eager to start. The infrastructure wasn't fully there, but it was enough for us to work with. We also had a great champion in the Director of the National AIDS Control Program. My good friend Joel, whom I first introduced you to in Rwanda, had been transferred to Côte d'Ivoire after his evacuation from Rwanda to serve as an adviser to the minister. He was critical in our success there as well. The ministry wanted to only distribute via their Central Medical Stores, or the Pharmacie de Santé Publique, which are essentially government-run pharmacies across the country. People were used to paying for medications at these pharmacies, which meant we received little pushback when they were asked to purchase these new HIV/AIDS medications. We also had the luxury of additional financial support from the French Solidarity Fund, which covered the cost for patients who couldn't afford the medication even at a discounted price. Through this centralized delivery system, we set up a system that linked the patient to the product, much like we did in Uganda.

In Vietnam, things weren't as simple.

The first issue we ran into was that the Ministry of Health didn't allow us to work with the private sector pharmacies to distribute the product. They also weren't interested in using the government-owned, public pharmacies because it would require the government to purchase the ARVs upfront, whereas the pilot intended for patients to pay for the treatment. We were stuck in a catch-22, and it took a long time to figure out what the actual issue was. Eventually, thanks to our partnership with a local professor, we learned that the government wasn't telling us that they were specifically interested in preventing transmission in mothers. Until this day, I don't know why they weren't more forthcoming with that information. Asian cultures tend to be less direct than American or European ones. Perhaps that's the reason, but the result, unfortunately, was that the pilot, as we intended it, never took off in Vietnam. Instead, they focused only on the prevention of mother-to-child transmission—a critical cause, but one that wouldn't allow for the same scale of intervention that we needed to prove that ARV distribution to the full population was possible.

Through it all, we worked to build a strong coalition between the companies, governments, and local implementers in every country. If these pilots were to scale up to countries around the world, we had to use them as an opportunity to build trust between these parties. Decisions were always transparent and reached with full consensus and with the buy-in of all parties involved, especially those in the country that would be most impacted by the interventions we were putting in place. Local champions played a critical role. Everyone was kept informed on progress and had a role in making any adjustments needed to improve the program. This type of coalition-building and championing often gets deprioritized in the face of significant logistical or political challenges, but the pilots taught me that it's one of the most critical building blocks of any sustainable public health intervention.

We also did our best to remove the public–private divide. You'll notice that in most countries we tried to introduce the pilot to, we were always faced with limitations around using private or public clinics and pharmacies. Shouldn't we be prioritizing by ability to deliver and not by sector? If you want to get your hair cut, you are going to go to the place that offers the best haircut. Why should public health be any different? We didn't always succeed—bureaucracy is a tough nut to crack, after all—but the successes we had in Uganda, Côte d'Ivoire, and Chile opened the door to a more effective way of distributing public health, some of which remain today.

In the end, to improve anything, we have to be willing to try and willing to fail. Doing the same thing, in the same way, over and over again knowing it doesn't work won't get us anywhere. Healthcare is no different. The mechanisms and systems we use to deliver care and treatment have to be willing and able to adjust to the changing needs of patients and our society as a whole.

The DAI pilots weren't just small-scale studies of ARV introductions in low- and middle-income countries. They were a proof-of-concept for an idea that had never been tried before. When we started, we didn't know exactly where we'd land, but we knew we had to try something different. Until HIV/AIDS, the idea of "access" was historically understood as a physical issue. Like the access you need to get into a special exhibit at your local museum. DAI was the first time access was used in the context of medicine. It wasn't just about getting medicines into the country. Access is not that simple. It was about actually getting them into people's stomachs—and doing that is much more complex than delivering boxes to a health facility. It's about enabling both treatment availability and accessibility. As we'll soon see, having both of those forces working together changes everything.

Despite the difficulties and pushback we faced with DAI, I stand behind the decisions we made and am incredibly proud of what was accomplished. DAI opened the door to better treatment access in low- and middle-income countries. A door that had been shut for far too long. I was eager to see who would walk through the door next.

Chapter 10

IT'S POSSIBLE!

It didn't take long for the pilot programs to create the demand and interest we hoped for. No country was just going to sit back and patiently wait their turn. Companies were going to have a hard time justifying not lowering costs for other countries when they already did for a few.

Even in the early days, the pilots had set up an irreversible dynamic: they have it in Uganda, we should have it here too!

One by one, before the pilots were completed, countries reached out asking how they could also receive ARVs. It was exactly what we hoped would happen. If you remember, through the French Solidarity Fund, France became the first country to give money to buy ARVs. The money first went to Côte d'Ivoire as part of DAI. The contribution showed that powerful governments like France did have a political interest in supporting HIV/AIDS drug access in low- and middle-income countries. The Fund, using the DAI model, soon began supporting additional countries, including Senegal, Zaire (now DRC), Congo, Cameroon, Guinea, Botswana, and Chad. And the demand spread to other parts of the world too, including Brazil, Colombia, and Mexico. I spent more time in an airplane than I did anywhere else that year.

In 1999, the CDC was requested to conduct an independent evaluation of the DAI pilots in Côte d'Ivoire and Uganda, led by two of my former partners in the PMTCT studies. Agence Nationale de Recherche sur le SIDA (ANRS/France) was requested to conduct the evaluations in Chile and Vietnam. The purpose of the evaluation was to determine if the pilots had met their objective of proving the feasibility of bringing ARVs to low- and middle-income countries in order to encourage investment and interest from funders.

We were in desperate need of some good news. In 1990, the World Health Organization estimated that roughly 8–10 million people were living with HIV/AIDS worldwide. By 2000, the HIV/AIDS epidemic had affected some 36.1 million people worldwide (cumulative), exceeding by 50 percent the best available 1991 projection made by WHO's Global Programme on AIDS. Of these, 95 percent lived in low- and middle-income countries, and there is reason to believe that an equally large percentage of them were unaware of their HIV status. An estimated 4 million people were newly infected in 2000, and 3 million died, bringing total deaths since the beginning of the epidemic to more than 16 million people.

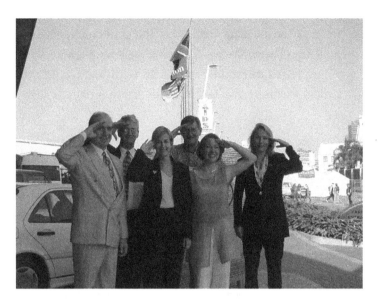

The team at the first AIDS conference in South Africa in 2000.

Thankfully, the results of the evaluation of the DAI pilots brought us the good news we so desperately needed. The findings were made public at the 2000 World AIDS Conference in Durban, South Africa. The 2000 World AIDS Conference wasn't just another conference. It was the first international AIDS conference in Africa—the continent most ravaged by the disease. It marked a significant milestone in the history of HIV/AIDS.

An 83-year-old Nelson Mandela spoke at the conference and said the following:

> No disrespect is intended towards the many other occasions where one has been privileged to speak, if I say that this is the one event where every word uttered, every gesture made, had to be measured against the effect it can and will have on the lives of millions of concrete, real human beings all over this continent and planet.

This is not an academic conference. This is, as I understand it, a gathering of human beings concerned about turning around one of the greatest threats humankind has faced, and certainly the greatest after the end of the great wars of the previous century.

...

We need, and there is increasing evidence of, African resolve to fight this war. Others will not save us if we do not primarily commit ourselves. Let us, however, not underestimate the resources required to conduct this battle. Partnership with the international community is vital. A constant theme in all our messages has been that in this inter-dependent and globalised world, we have indeed again become the keepers of our brother and sister. That cannot be more graphically the case than in the common fight against HIV/AIDS.[17]

During the week of July 9–14, 2000, 12,000 people from all over the world came together in Durban to mobilize the world's HIV/AIDS response. It had the world's attention. It was at that conference that HIV became the comparison point for public health—there's *before HIV* and *after HIV*. There have been other global pandemics; polio, for example. But HIV was unique in many ways. When it came along, we thought we were done with infectious diseases. HIV was also the first post-globalization pandemic. International media brought the plight of HIV/AIDS to living rooms around the world, and for the first time, we were being asked to care about an issue happening outside our own community.

---

17   Nelson Mandela, "Closing Address by Former President Nelson Mandela, XIII International AIDS Conference," Act Up, July 14, 2000, https://actupny.org/reports/durban-mandela.html.

So what did the evaluation of our DAI pilot programs find? The results were indisputable. ARV therapy could be safely and effectively used, even in the least developed countries. Patient adherence was similar to more developed countries and diversion of price-reduced drugs was limited. Not surprisingly, the evaluation also found that the price of the drugs was the main obstacle to expanding drug access in developing countries. Announcing these results at the World AIDS Conference opened the floodgates. Ours was the only tangible solution presented; everything else was a commitment to act with very little concrete action. To quote the head of UNAIDS, Peter Piot, "We have no excuse. We now know what to do and future generations will hold us accountable."

It was at this conference that Professor Jeffrey D. Sachs, then Chairman of the WHO Commission on Macroeconomics and Health, first called for a global fund to fight AIDS. He was echoed by many other leaders, including Peter. This recommendation was picked up the following year in the establishment of the Global Fund to Fight AIDS, TB, and Malaria.

At the same time, the cost debate roared louder than ever.

Before the DAI pilot showed that it was possible, there was no way that companies would have agreed to offer their medications at further discounted prices. But we hoped that by showing that ARV access was doable, we would have more negotiating grounds to push companies even further on price and volume.

The activists were also doing their part. I remember they would ask me which companies were giving me a hard time with negotiations. I hesitated at first, but eventually, I told them. They had built up incredible influence by that point of the pandemic, and truth be told, we needed all the help we could get. People were being infected at unbelievable rates, and after DAI, there was no more excuse for any manufacturer not to do their part.

Pharmaceutical companies—at the center of the world's attention and facing extreme pressure—eventually saw this as their opportunity to show the world that they weren't the big bad wolf they had been painted to be.

At first, they announced major infrastructure improvement investments.

Bristol-Myers announced a five-year donation of US $100 million to 160 programs to fight AIDS in Botswana, Namibia, Lesotho, Swaziland, South Africa, Burkina Faso, Côte d'Ivoire, Mali, and Senegal.

Merck and Gates Foundation would provide Botswana US $100 million over five years to support the country's National AIDS Coordinating Agency, strengthen infrastructure, and provide grants to community and faith-based organizations.

Abbott partnered with the government of Tanzania to modernize the country's public healthcare facilities and to improve services and access to care for people living with HIV/AIDS and other serious illnesses.

These are just a few of the examples. Each pharmaceutical company hoped the huge price tags behind these health infrastructures and system strengthening efforts would make the treatment pricing discussion go away. They didn't.

Boehringer Ingelheim, the manufacturer of Viramune (nevirapine), backed by the findings of the PMTCT study I told you about a few chapters back, was one of the first to announce a treatment-focused intervention. It planned to give nevirapine to Africa free for five years for use in blocking vertical transmission of HIV from infected pregnant women to their unborn children.

Soon after came Abbott Access, which broadened access to Abbott's HIV-care therapies in sixty-nine countries. Through Abbott Access, the company offered Kaletra and Norvir at a loss to Abbott. Abbott was the only pharmaceutical company to provide an HIV rapid test, Determine HIV, at no profit. In 2002, BI and Abbott partnered to offer Determine to PMTCT programs.

Merck also began donating its antiretroviral medicines to Botswana's national ARV therapy program and was the first to announce that it would sell its products in Africa at no profit. Gilead followed suit and launched the Gilead Access Program, which offered its once-daily medicines at a reduced price representing no profit to Gilead in sixty-eight countries (every country in Africa and in fifteen other countries designated as "least developed" by the United Nations).

Roche announced that it would not file patents on new HIV medications in low- and middle-income countries and would not take action against the sale or manufacture of generic versions of its HIV medicines. It also eventually made its two protease inhibitors available at no-profit prices to low- and middle-income countries.

Then came another major milestone for the pharmaceutical industry. The Accelerated Access Initiative (AAI) showed the shifting dynamic of pharmaceutical access for the developing world and the collaborative spirit of the time. Launched in May 2000 and driven by the companies involved with DAI, AAI involved seven pharmaceutical companies (Abbott, Boehringer Ingelheim, Bristol-Myers Squibb, Gilead Sciences, GlaxoSmith-Kline, Roche, and Merck & Co., Inc,) and five United Nations partners (UNAIDS, the World Health Organization, World Bank, UNICEF, and the United Nations Population Fund). The initiative was chaired by Jeff Sturchio, then head of public affairs at Merck.

Through AAI, ARVs were offered at about 10 percent of the commercial price to the public sector and non-governmental organizations that complied with specific conditions. The initiative started bearing fruit when funding mechanisms started to come into place in 2002. The market was now established. By the end of December 2006, more than 827,700 people living with HIV/AIDS in low- and middle-income countries were receiving treatment with at least one ARV medicine provided by the AAI companies.

Simply put, DAI kickstarted this momentum.

Through DAI we learned about the dynamics of sustainability and scalability. We learned that the entities invited to execute a program should be chosen based on demonstrated ability and capacity rather than on whether they're in the public sector or the private sector. We invited the public and private sectors to play in the same sandbox, and the results spoke for themselves. We learned about the value of promoting an entrepreneurial spirit, where countries are rewarded for doing well and companies are given the opportunity to profit. We learned how powerful it could be when the scientific community spoke with a single, unified voice. And finally, we learned how important it is to have champions willing to take risks, to try new things, and maybe even to fail. We didn't have the luxury to wait until all our Is were dotted and our Ts were crossed, but we moved forward anyway and that made all the difference. Just do it, and once you start seeing success, others will follow.

In the course of two years, DAI completely changed the HIV/ AIDS care and treatment landscape. It didn't reach millions of patients, but it did something that I'd argue was equally valuable. It broke the established standard of a single universal price and shattered the misbelief that the infrastructure of low- to middle-income countries could not support ARV distribution and administration. We created a model that prompted funding and support from around the world, helping more patients than one program ever could.

Chapter 11

A STORY FOR
THE AGES

After the Global Conference in Durban, things not only moved fast, but the scale of the response was unparalleled. The world was coming together behind one issue in a way we had never seen. Thanks to the DAI pilot programs, we had the proof of concept. We had media attention. We had a scientific community speaking in one voice. We had no more excuses.

Following Jeffrey Sachs's call for a global mechanism to fight AIDS in Durban, the Global Fund to Fight AIDS, Tuberculosis, and Malaria was officially announced in June 2001. The Fund intended to serve as a pooling mechanism for mostly public funding to support treatment and infrastructure improvements to accelerate the end of AIDS, tuberculosis, and malaria as epidemics.

The Global Fund's initial eighteen-member policy-setting board held its first meeting in January 2002 and issued its first call for proposals. By the time the Global Fund became operational, it had already received US $1.9 billion in pledges. In March 2002, a panel of international public health experts was named to begin reviewing project proposals that same month. In April 2002, the Global Fund awarded its first batch of grants—worth US $378 million—to thirty-one countries. From 2001 through 2018, the largest contributor by far has been the United States, followed by France, the United Kingdom, Germany, and Japan.

President Bill Clinton was a big reason the United States took the lead with the Global Fund. Multilateralism took a back seat, however—at least temporarily—when George W. Bush succeeded Clinton in January 2001.

At the G8 summit in Genoa in 2001, President Bush stood firm on the US's refusal of the Kyoto Protocol on global warming, saying it was bad for the US economy, and doubled down on its missile defense plan, deemed indispensable for American security. Little regard was shown by the impact of these decisions on other countries. In a 2001 letter to the European Union about the Global Fund, Robert Zoellick, the United States Trade Representative, expressed concern that "the sharing of drug pricing information can at times present problems under US antitrust laws."[18] The US had become increasingly reluctant to participate in collaborative, international initiatives at the expense of domestic practices—a move dubbed "cowboy diplomacy," referring to Bush's Texas roots.

---

18   Donald G. McNeil Jr., "U.S. at Odds with Europe Over Rules on World Drug Pricing," *New York Times*, July 20, 2001, https://www.nytimes.com/2001/07/20/world/us-at-odds-with-europe-over-rules-on-world-drug-pricing.html.

But Bush's cowboy diplomacy was shaken up by one of history's most significant events—September 11, 2001. That morning, the US awoke to four coordinated terrorist attacks by Al-Qaeda against the United States. Two planes flew into the upper floors of the North and South Towers of the World Trade Center in New York and a third plane flew into the Pentagon in Arlington, Virginia. After learning about the other attacks, passengers on the fourth hijacked plane, Flight 93, fought back, and the plane crashed into an empty field in western Pennsylvania about twenty minutes by air from Washington, DC. The attacks killed 2,977 people from 93 nations: 2,753 people were killed in New York; 184 people were killed at the Pentagon; and 40 people were killed on Flight 93.

The events of 9/11 showed the vulnerability of the United States and made it clear that national security—in a globalized world—required international collaboration.

It was in this environment that PEPFAR was born in 2002. The President's Emergency Plan For AIDS Relief was the United States Government's initiative to address the global HIV/AIDS epidemic. Unlike the Global Fund, it largely funded local NGOs. As of May 2020, PEPFAR has provided about US $90 billion in cumulative funding for HIV/AIDS treatment, prevention, and research since its inception, making it the largest global health program focused on a single disease in history—up until the COVID-19 crisis, that is. In addition to its public health objectives, you could say that PEPFAR became one of the first times that international aid was also utilized as a mechanism for maintaining national security. Continuous high infection rates were more likely to breed public dissatisfaction and unrest and potentially trigger security issues or terrorist activities that would threaten the United States. Plus, by providing financial support to address public health issues, the United States hoped to incite goodwill and build allies around the world.

Remember that just three years before during DAI discussions, US officials told me that contributing to HIV/AIDS treatment in developing countries was not on their agenda. What changed? In those three short years, those of us working in the HIV/AIDS space were able to create the perfect formula for policymaker buy-in: a clear threat with a clear solution and enough visibility to make them look good for solving the problem!

Global Fund and PEPFAR both provided ARVs to supported countries for free, which logically resulted in a rapid increase in treatment. But the huge scale of these interventions introduced a brand new problem: most country infrastructures were not prepared to handle the rapid increase. In the ideal situation, any changes would have been integrated into each country's existing system. This way, information and learnings would be retained. Unfortunately, because countries weren't prepared for this deluge of treatment, PEPFAR and Global Fund created what are known as parallel systems.

With DAI, we had to set up parallel systems too because it was a proof of concept and limited in scope. It wasn't what we wanted, but we did our best to set it up in a way that integrated existing mechanisms so learnings weren't lost. But in the case of PEPFAR and Global Fund, the aim was to ensure treatment was available and accessible in the long term to a large part of the population. To achieve that goal, avoiding parallel systems should have been a priority, but they didn't do it and chose short-term wins instead of long-term improvements. Integration is complex and time-consuming. It wasn't until ten years later that they tried to push for more integration, but by then, parallel systems were well established and made it very difficult to streamline.

To make matters worse, the new parallel systems were centrally managed by the donors themselves. This made it easier to provide technical and financial control, but also stifled local ownership and drive. For example, since the Global Fund was created, public sector contributions have constituted 95 percent of all financing raised; the remaining five percent comes from the private sector or other financing initiatives such as Product Red. The funds are also largely given only to the public sector (governments). By not engaging the private sector more significantly in the countries where funds are used, the Global Fund was essentially limiting the sustainability of their efforts. This is because private companies have a market incentive to do their best in order to increase profits. By doing their best, they improve local conditions and standards. Economic and social development go hand in hand with better healthcare. Without one, you can't have the other. However, market incentive to improve is not there in the public sector because funding is going to come in as they use it, regardless of how well they do in the process, or not. PEPFAR was set up in a similar way. Such funding models are built on a platform that allows countries little freedom and motivation to do better. As a result, there is little trickle-down effect to inform systemic change. Unfortunately, WHO, which was closely linked to the Global Fund, sees profit of any kind as a bad thing with no place in public health.

In the end, it shouldn't matter whether the money goes to the public or private sector. What should matter is how that money is expected to be used. If funders continue to dictate exactly how their money should be spent, versus seeing it as an investment to create a value chain that incentivizes improvement—for example, by paying local entities based on a percentage of goods distributed—countries will never stop being reliant on aid. It's a never-ending loop.

Despite the incredible amount of capital Global Fund and PEPFAR were able to pool, and the many millions of patients that they were able to help, we need to question whether they were designed effectively to make that money go as far as possible. Today, several African countries are no better off economically than they were after gaining independence from their European colonizers in the 1960s. In fact, Africa accounts for only a small percentage of the total world Global National Product (GNP), despite its abundance of natural resources.

* * *

Looking back at the HIV/AIDS epidemic, there is one question I often ask myself. Was our HIV/AIDS response a success?

I suppose it depends on how you define a success story. In the short term, we were able to move relatively fast, get the whole world behind one critical issue, and mobilize governments and companies to act. That's incredibly important, and we should never dismiss the significance of those achievements.

But for the sake of our future as a society, we have to look at whether we actually learned from HIV, and whether those learnings led to systemic changes. Could we prevent similar epidemics from happening again? COVID-19 has shown us otherwise. Many of the gaps I've described to you in this book so far remain. They may have changed or may be less significant, but unfortunately, they are very much still present.

During the peak of the HIV/AIDS epidemic, collaboration between countries and sectors was, I'd say, the primary driver of what we were able to accomplish. It was expected that this collaborative spirit would change and evolve with the changing geopolitical context, but in the face of a crisis like COVID-19, we should have known better. We know that together we are stronger, but today, political sovereignty supersedes public health. Few leaders were willing to take the road less traveled for fear of public backlash or losing control even if they knew it was for the greater good. As our collaborative spirit dissipated, we were also quick to forget just how important it is to have a unified scientific voice.

I recently listened to a podcast featuring former US CDC Director Nancy Messonier that provided some interesting perspective on this issue. Referring to the CDC's deliberation around recommending a third booster dose of the COVID-19 vaccine, Nancy said,

> The public is used to hearing scientists talk about settled science, and a lot of the disagreement and a scientific debate occurs behind the scenes. And what you're seeing now is that disagreement play out in real-time and us making decisions before all the science is settled. And I think that may be the new era going forward on this specific issue. CDC's advisory committee has to look at the data and interpret the data, but then use the data to make a recommendation. And there is inherently, in that step of analyzing the data and making a recommendation, a subjectivity to it. They have to take the data and pass it through their own values,

judgment, and experience. If it was purely a technical argument, frankly, you wouldn't need people. You could run it through a computer algorithm and have a result. And so the reason there is an advisory committee with experts is to try to balance out the difference between where the science says and where you have to make a judgment.[19]

I agree with Nancy on the pivotal role of scientific opinion because science is not black and white. What she is describing is what scientific leadership should be. The type of leadership that we sorely lacked during the COVID-19 pandemic. You have to make the call with the information that you have available, applying your best judgment and without fear of public backlash or repercussions. The implications of not making any call at all are much worse. Pascal taught me that in my earliest days as a physician. But consensus is important too. The scientific community should not be pressured to put everything out there without proper assessment and thought just because the rest of the world does—driven by the popularity of social media. As scientists, I think we have a responsibility to provide clarity. That is what science is meant for—to create the evidence that supports evidence-based decisions. Clarity comes from one clear consensus, not hundreds of scientific opinions. Early in a pandemic, we are never going to have all the science tied in a nice bow. More reason why we need consensus to align on the data we do have and the actions we need to take based on that information.

Unfortunately, there was no unified scientific voice during the

19   Nancy Messonnier, "Are Boosters Good Science—or Just Good Politics?" September 29, 2021, in *Today, Explained*, podcast, 37:14, https://podcasts.apple.com/au/podcast/are-boosters-good-science-or-just-good-politics/id1346207297?i=1000537032193.

COVID-19 pandemic to give policymakers a clear path forward. Other industries managed to collate a unified response. The G20 met. So did the G7. Central banks met and agreed on the need for a country-level stimulus package. The world's Ministries of Health didn't meet once to harmonize their policies and provide clear, consistent messages and guidelines. Worse, they met at the World Health Assembly in 2020, yet chose not to discuss it because it wasn't a dedicated COVID-19 meeting and the evidence was evolving. The world was at a standstill because of lockdowns, and they didn't discuss it because it wasn't on their agenda? Why didn't we see an urgent extraordinary meeting of scientists and policymakers convened by WHO to come to a consensus on a unified response?

During HIV, the scientific community was able to join together with one voice that clearly said, "We have studies to prove that access to antiretrovirals in low- and middle-income countries is feasible and it's a human right. We know that there will be challenges, but we are committed to figuring it out together. We must act now." We made it easy for decision makers, and they responded, putting in place policies that triggered funding and action. When the scientific community speaks loudly in one voice, politicians are less afraid to lead and act. In COVID-19, the world was bombarded with wildly disparate scientific opinions and very little fact.

With the lack of a global scientific consensus, each country announced individual rules and interventions with close to no global coordinated action, even though we were all dealing with the same virus. A virus that was clearly not observing borders and spreading across the world at an unprecedented pace. The result was an incalculable number of one-off local interventions that did little or came too late to stop a global virus. Instead, politicians were often left to make decisions based on unsubstantiated opinions and public pressure. We can see this in the haphazard way that measures were announced. In a matter of days, France and the UK changed their position from being staunchly against lockdowns to being for it. Why? They were receiving conflicting scientific opinions every day, and under growing public pressure, they chose to take the path most traveled and where they felt they'd face the least risk to their political standing.

To be fair, with HIV/AIDS, we had nearly two decades to learn and align, and a much more welcoming geopolitical environment. With COVID-19, we had weeks, but it doesn't explain the lack of leadership. At the time of writing this book, we are now two and half years into the pandemic and there is still no unified response, no scientific consensus. The fact is that while we didn't know everything about COVID-19 specifically, we know a lot already about how viruses behave, how they spread and mutate, and how populations react to public health measures. And we absolutely know what works and doesn't work when it comes to prevention. It's simple, really. General prevention doesn't work. Public health solutions that are targeted to the people most vulnerable to a disease do.

Our medicines supply chain is another gap that remains. Today, most supply chains for healthcare products, like medications, are still built and tracked around how many boxes are shipped and delivered, and not by how many patients receive and take the medication. How can you claim success if all you know is how many boxes arrived at your destination and not into the mouths of the patients who so desperately need them? With

DAI, we put systems in place that allowed us to link boxes of ARVs to patients. But once countries started scaling up, this practice didn't stick.

For example, the Accelerated Access Initiative (AAI) that I mentioned earlier didn't link boxes to patients. Why? Because putting in place the processes needed to track that kind of information at a large scale—especially in countries where there is little infrastructure to support it, is difficult, expensive, and time-consuming. I understand that sometimes you must focus on the short term given the urgency of the situation. I already told you about many times when I had to do the same. But that can't be the case when the short-term solution goes against the whole reason why you are doing something in the first place. The end goal was to help those with HIV/AIDS to live longer and more comfortably and to stop the spread of the disease. All the efforts to get companies to bring down their price, to transport these medications across oceans, to build up warehouses and distribution fleets to get them to clinics in some of the most remote corners of the world are for nothing if the patient isn't taking the medicine.

Eventually, WHO requested AAI to provide an update on the number of patients they were reaching. The companies involved with AAI didn't want to share their sales data with WHO, so AAI hired an external healthcare access consultancy, Axios International, which you'll hear more about soon, to help convert sales data to equivalent patient numbers. Using the sales data as a base, Axios estimated that between late 2000 and December 2003, more than 150,000 HIV patients in Africa received antiretroviral treatments through AAI. The data confirmed that, for the most part, the drugs were reaching the patients, which is great. But they also found another critical piece of information that brings us to my other point. Few patients were switching to second-line treatment. Second-line treatment is given when initial treatment (first-line therapy) doesn't work or stops working. On average, research showed that 25 percent of patients switched to second-line treatment after one year of treatment. This wasn't happening with many patients receiving treatments via AAI—making it clear that patients weren't taking their medication as prescribed or weren't followed up with properly.

Because patient numbers weren't tracked proactively, there was no way to know if patients were taking their medicine, how they were doing with it, or even if they were getting better or worse. That's because the structures in place then, and still to this day, don't allow us to properly track what patients are doing once they leave the hospital or clinic. Think about it. Once your doctor prescribes you a medication, you pick it up at the pharmacy and go home and hopefully take it as your doctor prescribed. You might have a follow-up appointment too, but if you cancel that, is that doctor's office going to stay on top of you until you reschedule or to make sure you are taking your medicine? The answer is no, even though today we have many digital systems or other complementary measures that should help us do this easily.

I remember when I visited a colleague and friend who had become the head of the Stop Tuberculosis Initiative at WHO. With HIV/AIDS, there was a resurgence of the tuberculosis (TB) epidemic because immunocompromised patients were more likely to develop serious TB infections and require a much longer treatment than people with normal immunity. If the treatment is not taken meticulously, the infection is not contained. Worse, resistant strains develop that are resistant to all existing anti-TB treatments. This means that patients—including those infected or not infected with HIV—are condemned to die if they catch such strains. The resistance was most prominent in South Africa, and there were serious concerns that it may spread further. Given the circumstances, it was important that patients take their full course of treatment. But as we said, the systems were not in place for that purpose. My colleague told me that the Stop TB Initiative had launched a pilot program to improve adherence to anti-TB treatment in which patients had to come to the TB health centers every morning to get their treatment. This way we could make sure that they were taking it consistently. My immediate reaction was, "Why don't we contact them instead to make sure they took it and visit them regularly?" He replied: "It would take significant resources and difficult logistics… Do you want to do this job?" We both laughed. I took it as a joke, but joking aside, his comment illustrated a much bigger issue—how we, the health experts, were incapable, or maybe unwilling, to look beyond hospitals or clinics for solutions. The initial results were promising, but over time, fewer and fewer patients came to the TB centers and the idea was dropped. Even if it succeeded, would we do the same for diabetics, and those with hypertension or heart disease? How many health centers are we going to build? And what for? Just to hand out medications?

COVID-19 provides a more current example of this same issue. The elderly or those living with chronic conditions were more vulnerable to COVID-19. Connecting with these patients to make sure they had the tools to avoid COVID-19 and the medications they needed to control their chronic conditions was critical. But we had few mechanisms to connect with them directly other than having their primary care physicians reach out one-by-one. At the scale of the pandemic, that wasn't feasible or easily replicable. For the most part, we had to wait for them to reach out to their doctors, or come to the hospital, which was already overwhelmed by COVID-19 patients. Instead of protecting them, these patients ended up in worse shape. Many were too afraid to go to the hospital for checkups or pharmacies for a refill of their medications, leading to a worsening of the chronic conditions they were already living with. Others unnecessarily lost their lives to COVID-19.

Our health system continues to be overly reliant on the hospital or clinic as the core provider of care. Most health systems don't have the infrastructure, the network, and the capacity to communicate with patients when they leave the hospital or the clinic. In the case of a pandemic, this made it very difficult to preemptively help vulnerable clusters prevent disease or to quickly identify and isolate the infected. The result is poor treatment adherence and less than optimal medical outcomes. This was obvious with HIV, yet we made the same mistake again with COVID-19.

And of course, last but certainly not least, one major area that has struggled to evolve since the HIV/AIDS pandemic is access to treatment.

After 1996, when non-nucleoside reverse transcriptase inhibitors became available, there was no other major treatment advance until 2012 when the US FDA approved the drug Truvada for pre-exposure prophylaxis, or PrEP. Why is that? Because of two factors: the introduction of generics and nonprofit pricing of branded drugs meant that companies no longer had a financial incentive to invest in research.

By the early 2000s, many companies—as part of their commitment to improving access to HIV medications—opened their patents or chose not to enforce them. Also, PEPFAR and the Global Fund created an attractive market for generics.

Plus, now that low- and middle-income countries had access to ARVs for several years, if a new branded ARV came along, it would largely be given to those with resistance to the existing ARVs. It usually takes several years for a patient to become resistant to a treatment, if at all. By the time the company developed sufficient sales in that country to make a profit, their patent would run out. This is why DAI had been designed to create a reasonably profitable environment for companies to ultimately help make it sustainable. The margins were significantly lower in DAI countries than developed countries due to the price difference, but companies still had a commercial incentive to keep providing the medication for the long term.

If they are making no profit at all via a nonprofit model, or potentially losing money by fully donating their stock, what is keeping them from pulling out of the arrangement? The answer should be because they are helping people. I agree. The companies did too, based on my conversations with them, but only to a certain extent, and only for so long. These are commercial ventures and have to provide value to their shareholders. We can discuss whether they should be or not, but the reality is that they are the only ones today creating the medicines patients need. The fact that they have an economic interest in doing so is one of the reasons we have these medicines at all. Standing by an idealistic view of free or very cheap medicines for all or refusing to work with the people who have the medicines will only slow us down and contribute to many lives lost. Access is so much more than free goods. Yet, low-price generics and donations continue to be thought of as the most effective solution to improve access to treatment in low- and middle-income countries.

After nearly a decade of intense focus on HIV/AIDS, the introduction of the Global Fund and PEPFAR signaled that we had solved the HIV problem, at least in the media's eyes. Little by little, you heard less about HIV. The scientists and researchers previously celebrated on television as heroes went back behind the curtain. Families ravaged by the disease disappeared from the front pages only to be replaced by the next topic du jour. With it, pharmaceutical companies stopped seeing the reputational value of their efforts and began to lose even more interest. You may be surprised to hear that in many developing countries, HIV/AIDS continues to be an issue to this day—but thankfully, is a much smaller one.

Every year, there are still 1.3 million estimated new infections worldwide. But it's not all bad.

In 2020, 37 million people were estimated to be living with HIV compared with 29 million in 2000. This is not because things have gotten worse, but because ARVs extended the life expectancy of patients significantly. Treatment turned it from a death sentence to a chronic disease. Out of 37 million people, 84 percent were estimated to know their HIV status, 73 percent had access to treatment and 66 percent had their viral load suppressed. HIV mortality also decreased by 60–80 percent in the past 20 years.

Those numbers signal huge improvements, and despite the gaps that remain, our global response to the HIV/AIDS pandemic marks a significant moment in history. There is a reason why every public health topic today is told through the lens of before or after HIV. HIV taught us what was possible. It taught us that viruses are much smarter than us and that in a globalized world, an issue 30,000 miles away can become everyone's issue overnight. It also taught us what we can achieve when we come together. Millions of people were saved because of the efforts of activists, companies, governments, researchers, scientists, and citizens who came together under one cause. That is why it's so important to reflect on why many of the learnings from HIV seem to have been forgotten. Many of the issues I've mentioned are systemic. They are so deep in the fabric of how we provide healthcare, some dating back as far as the tenth century, that it's almost impossible to imagine an alternative. If we keep doing the same thing and expecting different results, we are going to keep running into the same issues. As long as we ignore root causes, we are only compounding an already almost insurmountable challenge. My intention is not to minimize the significance of our achievements during the HIV era, but to remind us that we are, in fact, capable of better.

And where do I fit into all of this? In October 1999, just as our DAI pilots were wrapping up, I made a big decision to leave UNAIDS. The late '90s had brought a change to the organization. It started to become more bureaucratic, and every day there seemed to be a new hurdle put in place to slow down our progress. There were growing internal tensions between WHO and UNAIDS, and I wondered what that would mean for all the effort we had put in to stop the HIV/AIDS epidemic. It was a difficult decision. Why leave in the middle of the success you had worked so hard to create? I'm sure it sounds strange, but I had grown increasingly disillusioned with the public sector. You could say that after working so closely with both sides, it cemented my thinking that the private sector needed to have a bigger role in our public health response if we wanted to see any real systemic improvement. I had felt like this for quite some time. Maybe it's because I grew up in Lebanon where the public sector is extremely weak. Whatever the reason, these most recent experiences confirmed my thinking. I had also grown more concerned with the pharmaceutical industry's declining interest in access. We had worked so hard to get them to see the value of an investment in public health, and backtracking was unfathomable to me. If we could get pharmaceutical companies to start investing in access and seeing it as part of their business strategy, that would be a game-changer.

This was the first point in my life when I began to think more deeply about why the public and private sectors were so different. I couldn't point to one example when a government had driven long-lasting change. Not that day and not today. Look at two of the largest public sector initiatives of our lifetime, PEPFAR and Global Fund. So many billions of dollars. Did they help many people? Yes. But are those countries now able to protect their own populations from future health threats without external aid? No. You can look back as many years as you'd like, and it is always private industry driving progress. Even expeditions to the new world in the fifteenth century were funded by investors who expected a return on their investment.

HIV wasn't going to be our last pandemic, and other chronic and noncommunicable diseases like diabetes and cancer were starting to rear their ugly heads. The issue of access was here to stay. I've never been one to waste time, and I felt I could be much more useful working in and with the private sector. Turns out I wasn't going far.

Chapter 12

A NEW GENERATION OF HEALTHCARE ACCESS

"So you want pharmaceutical companies to pay you to help them reduce their drug prices? You are crazy." That's what former *Journal* reporter Mike Waldholz, who by now had become a friend, told me when I first mentioned the idea to him.

In 1997, that crazy idea gave birth to Axios International, a private healthcare consultancy based in Dublin, Ireland, with the mission to improve access to healthcare. Axios was founded by two Irishmen, Brian and John. You may remember Brian as the consultant who accompanied me and was instrumental in many of the negotiations with pharmaceutical companies during the early days of DAI. John was an accountant and a close friend of Brian's. Together, they started Axios to support me in the setup of DAI and to help pharmaceutical companies find ways to make their HIV products accessible across Africa and other low- and middle-income countries. In fact, under my UNAIDS capacity, I was their first client. In 1998, Brian and John were joined by Anne, a medical anthropologist who decided to give consulting a try after her UN contract ended. At the end of 1999, after leaving UNAIDS, I decided to join Axios as well. I told you I wasn't going far. Soon after, Peter from the Irish Development Authority came on board. So did Sowedi, the Ugandan pharmacist we had hired to run DAI in Uganda.

Today, private companies are not just applauded for, but are expected to be mission-driven. Social entrepreneurs, if you will. Investors specifically look for companies with a bigger purpose and clear social impact targets. That was not the case then, however.

Instead, there was a false misunderstanding that a for-profit, private company could not have a societal mission. The fact that Axios International was a for-profit company doing mission-based work seemed backward. To some, maybe even suspicious. Working with the private sector to accomplish public health goals was seen as a wild idea. There was no playbook for how to go about it, and many expected us to fail.

All of us involved in the early days of Axios knew we were taking a big risk. We were a unique bunch—a doctor, a pharmacist, a medical anthropologist, a business consultant, an accountant, and a development executive—but we had three important things in common. One was an entrepreneurial spirit. All of us had come from large organizations or companies and it was terribly exciting to be in this new world full of opportunities where we made the rules.

Axios couldn't have been more different than WHO and the UN. There were only six of us to drive the work with a small staff to support us. We couldn't pass anything off or spend days discussing alternatives. There was no endless paperwork or bureaucracy to get things done. We decided on a path forward and put the wheels in motion to implement it. I had taken a big salary cut by joining Axios and the perks that came with working for the UN were long gone, but the freedom to think and act outside the box was liberating and exciting. It had been a long time since I felt that way. Probably since I first arrived in Paris from Lebanon thirteen years earlier.

We also all believed strongly in our mission to improve access to healthcare in low- and middle-income countries. We didn't want to just come up with ideas and pass them off to someone else to implement or write endless reports on what should be done. We wanted to go out there and do it.

This brings me to my third point. Beyond our roles as professionals working in the healthcare field, we were also people. We saw firsthand the incredible suffering that HIV/AIDS was placing on the world and felt a calling to make it better. I don't know if we realized it at the time, but the six of us shared a critical belief that is at the heart of the organization to this day: change comes from a willingness to do things differently. It was hard, uncomfortable, and even scary at times, but we believed there was a better way. We also trusted, perhaps naïvely, our ability to get us there.

It was a mission I had dedicated the last ten years of my life to and one I had every intention of continuing. Getting sick in many of these countries was a death sentence. Our intention was to change that reality so that whether you were born in Africa or the United States, you knew there was hope. We wanted to change what it meant to be a patient in one of these countries. And that involved more than just providing medications for the short term.

From what I had seen over the last decade, and even as a young man in Lebanon, I felt the quickest, most effective way to get there was by working with private companies or any institution ready to roll up their sleeves and do the work. The intention was not to leave out governments completely but to leverage the market forces that drove private sector investment in order to expedite the response to critical public health needs. There was no reason to be limited to the public sector only. We had shown that through DAI, but we soon had another chance through the Viramune (nevirapine) Donation Program (VDP).

Following the AIDS conference in Durban, Boehringer Ingelheim (BI) contacted Axios for help managing the commitment it had made during the conference. Driven by the success of DAI, several pharmaceutical companies had pledged their support through medicine donations or infrastructure improvements. Low- and middle-income countries, especially those in Africa, were a new world for most of these companies, and many were anxiously seeking partners to help bring their pledges to life.

BI had announced that it would provide its drug, nevirapine, free of charge to developing countries for use in the prevention of mother-to-child transmission of HIV during delivery. Nevirapine might ring a bell for you. A few chapters back, I told you about the controversial clinical trial working group I led which found that a single tablet of nevirapine administered to a woman just prior to giving birth and a small dose of a syrup version of the drug given immediately to the newborn can significantly reduce the risk of transmission to the child. The BI donation meant the drug would finally be getting to pregnant mothers in need. Or at least, that was the intention.

BI had begun shipping nevirapine to countries around the world soon after their announcement in Durban. A year later, I saw the BI team at another conference and they shared with me that BI was growing increasingly frustrated that few countries or health programs had taken advantage of the offer. Mother-to-child transmission of HIV accounted for many new HIV infections, so why weren't countries jumping all over this offer? The answer is that price is just one of many factors that stand in the way of access.

The first issue was that donations were first only made available to governments, which significantly limited the reach of the donation. The expectation was that the government would be responsible for distributing it throughout the country, but that didn't happen. Despite the incredible need for these medications, most of these countries didn't have the experience managing a donation like this, and the project got stuck in bureaucratic approvals and processes. There was little precedent for how to manage large quantities of more specialized medications like nevirapine. Most of their experience was with primary care medication, like aspirin, which doesn't require the same kind of experience and oversight to manage. How and where would they store nevirapine? How would they distribute it to pregnant women, and how would they forecast the quantity of products needed? How would they identify pregnant women that needed it? These were just some of the questions they had, and unfortunately, in the beginning, there were no answers. The companies, used to operating in more developed environments, were working under the assumption that providing the medication free or at a low cost was sufficient. They all learned quickly that it wasn't.

BI hired Axios to increase the number of countries benefiting from VDP—a relationship that continued for thirteen years. We first set up an application-and-review process to help organize the distribution of the supply of the drugs. Working off the lessons learned from DAI, we opened up the program to any institution able to receive, store, and administer nevirapine to pregnant women, based on pre-established criteria. This included governments, nonprofit organizations, and private clinics. We got a lot of pushback on this. Many, perhaps most, thought public health should be a government-only concern. While institutions needed sign-off from the country's Ministry of Health to participate, all organizations that met the required criteria were welcome to apply.

We also reached out to anyone and everyone to let them know about VDP. We learned from our first round of outreach that many had no idea the program even existed, let alone that they could receive nevirapine free-of-charge. Sometimes it's the most obvious, simple steps that make all the difference.

Once nevirapine arrived in the country, our Axios project manager worked closely with each implementing institution to manage available stock and support patient follow-up. We incorporated a long list of practices I learned back in my DAI days. Forms were developed to facilitate supply forecasting and patient follow-up, and institutions were responsible for completing them on an ongoing basis. All drug forecasts were based on actual patient usage, and institutions were expected to track patient-level data and report back to us. This helped to make sure that the medicine was actually getting to the patients who needed it.

My wife, Marie-Helene, had joined Axios as our seventh employee. She became the main manager of VDP, including monitoring the forms for accuracy. But the responsibility for doing good work was on the recipient of the donation. We visited from time to time, but if they wanted to keep receiving the medications, they had to complete the forms accurately and in a timely manner. In turn, that helped build their capacity for drug and supply chain management.

By allowing all types of organizations to participate, the approach we used with VDP removed unnecessary barriers that made governments the sole providers. Instead, our approach encouraged entrepreneurship and creative thinking. Any organization that wanted to participate had a chance to do it. Those that didn't meet the minimum criteria were encouraged and provided with recommendations to increase their capacity in order to participate in the program, helping to improve overall local capacity for management of HIV/AIDS patients. As you might expect, in the beginning, we did get pushback from governments as well as some academics who felt like public health was the domain of government. But public health belongs to the people. Over time, as the program became successful and governments began to receive international praise for their efforts to assist HIV-positive mothers, they eventually dropped their resistance.

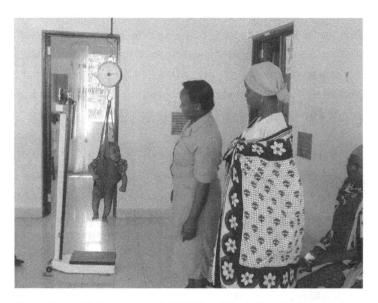

A baby getting weighed by a nurse at a health facility in Tanzania. His mother had received treatment through the Viramune Donation Program to help prevent mother-to-child transmission of HIV/AIDS.

VDP provided nevirapine at no cost to 2.3 million mother–child pairs in sixty countries for eleven years (between 2000 and 2011). It also triggered several operational and policy-level changes at the country level. VDP helped countries expand PMTCT services, improve their logistics capacity, and increase social support mechanisms for HIV-positive pregnant women. Importantly, it mobilized new PMTCT policies, which opened the door to new donor funding and partnerships with national and international organizations. We also found that NGOs and private organizations were able to start implementing the program faster than other kinds of participating institutions. Later came larger organizations, and eventually the government. Once governments got on board, the number of patients escalated quickly across institutions. This increased our confidence that we were on the right path with our multisectoral approach. Start first with NGOs and private institutions who are willing to move quickly, then use them as a proof of concept to get governments on board. You need governments to scale, but you don't need them to start. Start with what you have and the rest will come.

I remember the words Tanzania's former Minister of Health told me: "It was like rain when it was so dry. Once nevirapine was available to mothers, the government was encouraged to put new PMTCT policies in place, and once we did, so many organizations who were originally hesitant to work with us came to our aid." Her leadership was a key reason why we were so successful in Tanzania in the early days of Axios. She was open to new ideas and always willing to try a different way, if the usual way wasn't working. Having that kind of champion on our side made all the difference.

Ultimately, VDP acted as a catalyst for systemic changes at the institutional and national levels. Those changes were primarily driven by one thing—the availability of treatment. We saw this with DAI before, and VDP was no different. Treatment gave people hope, and that hope drove action—from the top and from the bottom. Today, VDP has become a model for how private, pharmaceutical initiatives can impact capacity and foster diverse public–private partnerships among government, companies, local institutions, and international NGOs to facilitate sustainable improvements. Over the coming years, Axios would replicate the VDP model time and time again across different types of access programs, not just donation programs. You'll hear more about that shortly.

* * *

In addition to BI, there were several other pharmaceutical companies struggling with the reality of working in Africa. Many were in the same boat. Huge investments had been made in the region with little knowledge of what it took to turn those investments into results. Working in developing nations was so different from the industrialized world these companies were used to. One of those struggling companies was Abbott.

You may remember that my relationship with Abbott began a few years earlier. I had met with their then CEO to try to get them to offer their ARV, called Norvir, as part of DAI. Once I joined Axios, I reached out again to their head of public affairs. They had just decided to do what their peers did (i.e., invest millions of dollars in Africa to fight against HIV/AIDS), and I knew they would need help.

Part of that investment was Abbott's Access to HIV Care access program, which made Norvir and their rapid HIV tests available at a nonprofit price with no markup. Yet Abbott was worried about product diversion. BMS and Glaxo-Wellcome were having significant diversion issues after launching their own access initiatives and finding their discounted products being sold on black markets from Germany to the UK. Both companies were using typical sales channels to sell their drugs at significantly discounted prices in lower income countries. There was no mechanism to assess whether these sales points were tracking whether the patients receiving or purchasing the drugs were actually using them. As a result, many of the drugs were being mailed to the EU and sold for much, much higher prices. Using what Axios had learned from VDP, we worked with Abbott to implement a centralized mechanism for selecting qualified institutions to receive the ARVs and tests, and to improve the capacity of local institutions to manage products and prevent drug diversion. The mechanism put in place a strong foundation that helped the program eventually reach more than six million patients in sixty-nine countries.

The risk and size of Abbott's investment and its potential reputational impact meant that senior executives were paying close attention to what was happening on the ground. In 2001, Abbott had begun donating their rapid HIV tests to support our efforts in preventing mother-to-child transmission of HIV/AIDS in Tanzania, and their CEO was eager to visit Tanzania to see the work firsthand. Today, you rarely hear about CEOs making trips to Africa or any other less-developed regions. Their priorities have shifted, but in the early 2000s, after several rough years of being dragged in the mud for not lowering their prices, pharmaceutical CEOs were eager to show their commitment to the region. I suspect there was a good deal of curiosity too. This part of the world had never crossed their radar in the past. There was no commercial market in these countries due to affordability issues, and before HIV, no one was pushing these companies to look beyond profit. But now, deep into the HIV/AIDS epidemic, there was no going back. The entire world was paying attention to what they were doing, and they would need to figure out how to make their treatments available for the long term—for HIV and other diseases.

It took six months to establish the proper security apparatus in Africa and to get everything planned. It was a huge deal to have such a big name make the trip. At Axios, we were excited to have the opportunity to show him the issues firsthand. Hearing about it and seeing it in person are very different things, and we hoped his visit would result in big changes for Tanzania. He was scheduled to arrive on September 15, 2001, but his trip was delayed as a result of the September 11 attacks in the United States. Thankfully, a year later, he was able to make the trip.

He had never been to Africa. I asked him why he decided to come. He told me that the world was changing and that Abbott had an obligation to address it. But to do that, he needed to understand these changes better. We took him to a remote village in the Rungwe district of Tanzania. We met with the Tanzanian president and Minister of Health. Over one week, we took him all around the country. One of our stops was at Muhimbili National Hospital in Dar es Salam, Tanzania. Muhimbili was intended to serve as a referral hospital for specialty care and complicated cases. In other words, this is where sick patients from around the country were supposed to be sent for more specialized care. Yet after decades of chronic underfunding, the hospital's systems, technical capacity, and infrastructure had deteriorated to the point of dysfunction.

Sick patients lined the hallways. Waiting rooms were filled to capacity with sick, exhausted people who had walked for hours, perhaps days to get there, only to wait several more hours to be seen by the few doctors on duty. Once they were seen by a doctor, the treatments available to them were rudimentary at best. For those used to hospitals in Europe and the US, it was hard to wrap your head around such a scene. He wasn't much of a talker, but since it was his first time in Africa, I can only guess what he was feeling based on how I felt the first time I saw it. I never imagined that such a reality still existed in the world. But it very much did across every corner of Africa.

He kept silent for quite a while. I started to wonder if we had done something wrong or not met his expectations somehow. As we walked back to the car, after what felt like hours of silence, he asked me what it would take to fix it. I didn't know what to expect from his visit, but I certainly wasn't expecting Abbott to commit even more money. Pharmaceutical companies were under extreme public pressure to address the HIV/AIDS pandemic. Until then, they were mostly under the radar, manufacturing and selling their drugs with little fanfare. But HIV/AIDS changed all of that, and Muhimbili provided a concrete, physical example to show the world.

I promised to come back to him with a budget. A month later, I met him in Chicago with a one-page, US $10 million budget for the first year. He approved it on that day, kickstarting a multi-year journey to modernize Muhimbili. Can you imagine any government signing a US $10 million dollar deal in one day? If this was the public sector, we would have been waiting for months, if not years.

Muhimbili National Hospital was a large hospital serving a significant part of Tanzania—it employed more than 2,500 people and there were over 1,000 beds. But the equipment was poor, there were few qualified doctors, and overcrowding was rampant. Patients who should have been getting care and treatment for everyday ailments at their local health facility were instead going to Muhimbili because standards were so bad elsewhere—this led to overcrowding and prevented the hospital from focusing their resources on specialized care.

Thanks to the CEO's commitment, Abbott's donation, and the support of the Minister of Health, a new three-story, 3,700–square meter outpatient treatment department was constructed, state-of-the-art laboratory equipment was installed (resulting in one of the most advanced laboratories in Africa), and general management, IT, human resources, and other support systems were overhauled. The outpatient department included thirty-four patient examination rooms, a pharmacy, and training facilities for medical students and healthcare professionals. Laboratory capacity significantly increased too. The average number of chemistry diagnostic tests processed in a day, for example, increased from 75 to 8,000 tests. We also put in place a medical record system that kept all details for one patient in one file. Until then, there was a new medical record created for every time a patient went to the hospital, making it impossible to track a patient's history. The new system was a game-changer.

When we first started the project, we knew we would need to bring someone on board who was an expert in hospital management. I remembered that one of the case studies I had read while doing the executive training at INSEAD talked about how the CEO of Karolinska Hospital in Sweden had completely revolutionized a hospital. It was a long shot, but I decided to give him a call to see if he'd be interested in helping us. Much to my surprise, he said yes. Thanks to him, we were able to implement the new patient record system, but many of the other improvements we hoped to put in place never came to fruition due to bureaucratic issues. As it was a public hospital, every change and improvement we made at Muhimbili had to be reviewed by the Tanzanian parliament. With the support of several champions in Tanzania's government, we were able to get some of our ideas approved, but even with their passion and commitment, the bureaucracy of the public sector was too much to overcome. For example, the hospital employed 2,500 people. Much more than was necessary. But we weren't able to let anyone go because they were government employees, rendering many of our recommendations obsolete.

Many great ideas never saw the light of day in Tanzania. Why? Because the healthcare systems in Africa and many low- and middle-income countries are almost exclusively dependent on and controlled by the public sector—a sector that has proven slow to react to societal changes, creating a rigid healthcare system exceptionally resistant to reform.

This—and many of my early experiences with Axios—cemented my belief in the limitations of the public sector and the importance of multi-stakeholder, multi-sector collaboration.

Chapter 13

BREAKING BARRIERS

While we largely succeeded in expanding Muhimbili's capacity for specialized treatment, it was one hospital—often thousands of miles away from many of Tanzania's residents. If Muhimbili National Hospital was to fulfill its mandate as a specialized hospital, we needed to improve healthcare delivery within local communities too.

But how could we do that? We couldn't magically manifest and train a whole new generation of health providers overnight, or properly stock every health facility in the country with functioning, state-of-the-art equipment and critical medicines. At least, not in the short term.

I've talked a lot already about the difference between short- and long-term solutions. In a public health crisis, like HIV and COVID-19, urgency is paramount. We don't have the luxury of spending months and years discussing how to implement complicated, complex solutions that will change the very essence of a country's health system. While those may be helpful in the long-term, it's not always practical and will undoubtedly contribute to many lives lost in the short-term. Public health experts tend to focus on the best solution, but sometimes, when lives are at stake, we need to focus on what is adequate and fast.

Putting in place a shorter-term response doesn't mean ignoring the long-term solution. They can be done simultaneously. Start by identifying solutions that can be implemented quickly within the existing infrastructure and resources available in the country, and support local capacity building so the solution can be maintained even if the original funders pull out of the project. Axios knew that many of these commitments by the pharmaceutical companies wouldn't last forever. That's why we always set up our programs in a way that would mobilize local organizations to take it over when the time came, or prompt system-wide improvements through policy change. We often chose to take a modest approach, implementing simple but significant improvements that they could maintain on their own, even if funding was decreased. We also looked for untapped, alternative approaches living within the existing healthcare ecosystem.

Here's an example from Tanzania. As you already know, mother-to-child transmission of HIV accounted for many new HIV infections in Africa, and Tanzania was no different. Through VDP, nevirapine was available to pregnant women and their babies to minimize the chance of transmission. But at first, the medication was out of reach for many mothers delivering at home in rural areas. The drug is meant to be given at medical facilities, but in Tanzania, more than 50 percent of pregnant women delivered outside their hospital or clinic. We had a big issue on our hands.

Instead of going to the closest hospital or health facility, traditional birth attendants, or TBAs, often helped pregnant women deliver at home. TBAs were local village women who had delivered hundreds of babies in their lifetime, often taught by their own mothers. TBAs would go to the woman's house when it was time to deliver. They weren't "qualified" health providers with traditional schooling, but the TBAs I met were skilled and had delivered more babies than your average gynecologist. They played a central role in healthcare delivery in these rural settings.

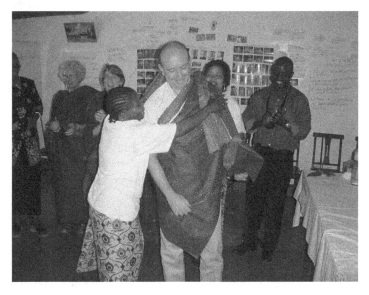

Receiving a gift from a Traditional Birth Attendant in Kilombero District, Tanzania. TBAs were eager to help prevent mother-to-child transmission of HIV/AIDS in their villages.

To address the issue of home delivery, Axios first decentralized the availability of nevirapine by expanding its distribution to include dispensaries in rural areas, not just large hospitals. Second, we wanted to mobilize TBAs to help improve the use of nevirapine in these regions. To do it, we would train them to raise community awareness of PMTCT, refer pregnant women to the formal health system, and provide psychosocial and nutrition counseling to HIV-positive pregnant women. In the case of HIV-positive women who lived far from health facilities, they would be given a nevirapine tablet during antenatal care and the TBA's role was to remind the woman to take her tablet during labor. The next day TBAs would accompany the mother and baby to the health facility so that health center staff could administer the nevirapine dose to the baby. Our main goal was to have TBAs serve as champions to encourage women to get tested for HIV/AIDS and to deliver in health facilities where there were more resources and expertise to address complications. In the short term, we also hoped training TBAs to encourage women delivering at home to take nevirapine would help to lower PMTCT rates.

Sounds like a good plan, right? The Tanzania Ministry of Health didn't think so, at least at first. "They aren't medically qualified providers!" they said. True, they weren't. But there was a severe shortage of medical providers in Tanzania and around the continent. TBAs were already a central, accepted part of a pregnant woman's health journey in these villages. Should pregnant women continue to suffer until we were able to get more doctors and nurses into these villages? Does it really take a medical degree to give a woman a pill? I don't blame them for thinking the way they did. It's another example of the health system's rigidity. They were trained to think that way. Just like I was. And my colleagues at Bichat-Claude were similarly trained when they removed Pascal from all his medications. And so were the accomplished researchers when they refused to accept the placebo option in the PMTCT clinical studies.

We ran into a similar issue with Abbott's voluntary counseling and testing (VCT) program. VCT had become more popular once treatment options became available in Africa. People were much more willing to get tested now that they knew there was something to help them if they tested positive. An HIV test typically involved a quick finger prick to draw blood. Although anyone can prick a finger, in Tanzania, only lab technicians were allowed to do it. But in some districts of Tanzania, like Rungwe, there were only two lab techs for more than 250,000 people. What if we allowed nurses and other health workers at health facilities to do the finger prick as well? That would significantly lessen the load on lab technicians and increase the number of people getting tested. I remember talking to the head of the lab at Muhimbili, whom I had met and befriended when he served as a researcher in one of the PMTCT studies several years earlier. He was vehemently opposed to having others do the finger prick. "It's a lab technician's job to carry out a diagnostic test," he said. The Ministry of Health agreed with him. It didn't come easy, but eventually, we convinced them. I'm sure you won't be surprised to hear by this point that we did it by doing a pilot project. Once we told policymakers it was just a pilot, the unnecessary barriers they had put up came down quickly. It makes you question how important those barriers were in the first place if they can come down so quickly at the simple suggestion of a pilot versus a permanent solution.

Most policymakers are scared to risk doing things differently, even if they know that different can be better—that's the real barrier, not their concern for having women receive a pill from a non-medical provider, or having their finger pricked by a nurse. Doing things differently can result in failure, which in turn can lessen their chance of reelection or promotion. It can mean criticism from their peers or losing their jobs. Why take a risk if you are going to get paid regardless? With a pilot, the potential political implications and level of risk are much less significant. It was just a pilot, after all…

In 2005, in collaboration with the government of Tanzania and the Elizabeth Glaser Pediatric AIDS Foundation, the pilot began in two hard-to-reach districts of Tanzania, Hai and Kilombero. The pilot made available both BI's nevirapine and Abbott's Determine rapid HIV tests in hard-to-reach areas by mobilizing TBAs and local health facilities. With the help of the TBAs, the number of women getting tested and delivering in health facilities continuously increased throughout the implementation of the pilot. The Axios project in the two districts accounted for 80 percent of pregnant women tested for HIV. As expected, TBAs went above and beyond in their role. Some even wrote a song that they would perform at the weekly market to increase awareness of testing and the options available to women at delivery. They also formed a social support group for mothers who tested HIV-positive.

In 2006, the pilot was handed over to the district health authorities in a smooth transition. The Ministry of Health adopted TBA training guidelines, and the president of Tanzania at the time publicly advocated the use of TBAs. The results of the pilot illustrate how short-term solutions like pilots can help drive policy changes and sustainable improvements in a country. It also highlights the benefits of looking for alternate solutions to complement the traditional health system—in other words, "thinking beyond the hospital." A hospital or clinic is one place where care can be provided, but it's not the only one. There are many other parties, like TBAs, that can help when a hospital can't be reached or is overwhelmed. An overreliance on hospitals, as I've mentioned many times already, is an outdated way of thinking about healthcare. There's a whole world outside hospitals and clinics that we should be tapping into to better care for patients.

In the end, what we tried to do in Tanzania and around the world through the Viramune Donation Program and Abbott's Access to HIV Care program was simple. We identified the hurdles causing the problem and found new ways to overcome them, quickly. We didn't keep doing the same thing repeatedly hoping for a different result. That's the definition of insanity, right?

I don't mean to suggest that governments are insane. I do mean to suggest that my experience with governments during these early days of Axios, and even earlier with UNAIDS and WHO, strengthened my resolve to mobilize the private sector to expedite and facilitate public health interventions. While many governments eventually came around, the blatant inflexibility several showed along the way severely stunted our progress and limited the impact of many of these interventions. The health infrastructure in many low- and middle-income countries at that point was almost entirely controlled by the public sector, and without their willingness to think outside the box and collaborate with non-public partners, there was a limit to what could be accomplished. The incredible work of forward-looking public sector leaders like the Minister of Health in Tanzania, and others like her, were no match for an inflexible, antiquated healthcare system that refused to change.

For example, Axios was hired to evaluate two separate pharmaceutical companies' programs in Africa. Both programs had lofty goals and they certainly succeeded in improving access to treatment and building select infrastructure, but neither succeeded in changing the fabric of how HIV/AIDS care and treatment were delivered in Africa. These programs were built in a vertical, top-down fashion much like those of large international donors. What that meant is that companies, in hope of avoiding price cuts, donated millions and millions of dollars in areas where they felt there was a need to strengthen infrastructure and provide care. There was little consultation with country leaders or collaboration to identify real areas of need. Beyond PR events where Ministers of Health were photographed with CEOs, behind the scenes, companies decided where to put the money and countries took what they could get. We saw new hospitals built and millions of people receiving treatment. But what happened when the money ran out? Did the country have the means and experience to run those hospitals, or to purchase these drugs on their own for the population? These programs were largely a short-term band-aid on a much deeper, bleeding wound.

Some may say that the problem was that there wasn't sufficient investment from the private sector, not that the public sector held back progress. But funding is not the only issue. Just look at PEPFAR, the largest commitment by any nation to address a single disease in the world. From 2001 to March 2021, PEPFAR supported antiretroviral treatment for nearly 18.2 million people with an investment of US $90 billion. That's about US $5,000 per person (when the cost of treatment is only a couple of hundred). In comparison, Tanzania's per capita GDP is around US $1,000. Much of the cost per patient was driven by the operating costs of US-based NGOs running these programs.

In other words, a significant percentage of the money being pumped into Africa to support these patients was ultimately going back into American coffers. The same is true for public donor interventions from other countries.

But is this the only way? It's not.

In addition to giving patients treatment, PEPFAR could have been designed to promote longer-term social and economic development. For example, instead of donating treatment directly to the government for public distribution, they could have reimbursed hospitals for the cost of treatment, enabling them to use those funds to upgrade their facilities. Or donors could pay hospitals and health facilities for the cost of treatment for each patient based on predetermined criteria. If health facilities wanted to have and keep free treatment for their patients, they would be encouraged to use the money to improve their capacity and infrastructure. This is a classical model used by social security systems and insurance schemes in many countries. Medical interventions and medications are reimbursed per patient, prompting health facilities to continuously improve their capacity and ensure that patients are satisfied.

Instead, when discussing their donations or grants, donors often speak about "burn rate," or how much and how quickly money is being spent. What they should be talking about is return on investment. While there is accountability for money spent and number of patients reached in the short term, there is no obligation for long-term impact built into most donor programs. Donors decide how the money should be spent and local governments or NGOs implement that request. During COVID-19, governments had no issue giving individuals and businesses money to kickstart their finances. But they won't do the same for international aid because the truth is that aid is a mechanism for control. By keeping countries dependent on their aid, donor governments are able to indirectly influence national decisions to their benefit.

Here's another way donor funding can be used more effectively. The head of WHO's Roll Back Malaria Initiative used Global Fund money in a new way—to subsidize malaria treatment. The government bought malaria treatment from manufacturers at a lower price. Global Fund funding was used to cover the bulk of that cost and local distributors paid the rest. They then sold it to the patient with a small enough markup that the patient could afford, while still making a little money for the distributor in the country. In other words, she used the market-driven model for medication supply chain and dispensation utilized in richer, more developed countries. In the past, malaria drugs were simply purchased and given to the Central Medical Store for distribution, yet her idea was ingrained in economic development. By subsidizing the cost of treatment, she favored market dynamics and stimulated the local economy while addressing patient needs, much like PSI did with social marketing of condoms during the HIV pandemic. Unfortunately, because of donors' opposition, it didn't last long. It took away some of the power from the government and distributed it to local wholesalers. That's what they didn't like.

If more solutions like this were put in place, there would have been no need for PEPFAR to spend anywhere near US $5,000 per person and the GDP in many of these countries may have increased. Instead, they created a mechanism that has made countries entirely reliant on their aid and an environment that actually discourages innovation and initiative and encourages corruption.

In the book *Dead Aid,* former World Bank consultant Dambisa Moyo calls the aid industry both ineffective and "malignant." She says that "by thwarting accountability mechanisms, encouraging rent-seeking behavior, siphoning away talent, and removing pressures to reform inefficient policies and institutions," aid weakens social capital and ensures countries remain poor. That is exactly what happened during the HIV/AIDS epidemic. Moyo tells us that "between 1970 and 1998, when aid flows to Africa were at their peak, poverty in Africa rose from 11 percent to a staggering 66 percent."

Instead, she proposes a new way forward. "What if, one by one, African countries each received a phone call, telling them that in exactly five years the aid taps would be shut off—permanently?"[20] Countries would have no choice but to use alternative financing mechanisms beyond aid, like increased trade among African nations and emerging markets, foreign direct investment, and microfinance.

The reality is that even when the public sector tries to innovate, the result is often a big, clunky, political monster that costs millions (or, in PEPFAR's case, billions) to implement. They aren't typically agile and results-driven. Innovation is driven by risk. You can't have one without the other.

Does this mean that governments should not play a role in public health? Absolutely not. They have a critical role to play.

20 Dambisa Moyo, *Dead Aid: Why Aid Is Not Working and How There Is a Better Way for Africa* (New York: Farrar, Straus and Giroux, 2009), 144.

Governments should serve as regulators to ensure that patients are getting the best standard of care and, when possible, finance healthcare by reimbursing services from both the public and private sectors. With the world evolving like it is today, we are going to need a balance of public and private healthcare interventions if we want to improve healthcare for the greatest number of people. Governments don't need to be the only ones to provide care. Instead they need to be willing to finance whoever is ready to provide the service—if that happens to be the private sector and not the public, that should not be a barrier. Notice that I said they need to reimburse healthcare services, not just treatments. That idea, called value-based care, is a payment model that offers financial incentives to physicians, hospitals, medical groups, and other healthcare providers for meeting certain performance measures. If hospitals provide a good service and their patients are getting a good outcome, they get paid. Just like the economic development model we discussed above, value-based care encourages entrepreneurship and development of the sector, and that's exactly what we need—in developing and developed countries alike. Sounds logical, right?

Essentially, governments should encourage collaboration and innovation by inviting partners across the spectrum to work together toward the common goal of better healthcare. Being a regulator doesn't mean being a barrier. It means ensuring a quality standard of care. They should encourage multi-sector investment in healthcare to meet public health priorities and put policies in place to scale up these interventions once they are shown to be successful. They should push for quality, sustainable public health solutions and away from overreliance on international aid.

Meanwhile, the difficulty in working with governments in these early projects pushed pharmaceutical companies further and further away from HIV/AIDS. In their place came public initiatives like PEPFAR and Global Fund, which, despite their success in bringing treatment to millions of people, significantly contributed to economic stagnation in many low- and middle-income countries. Pharmaceutical companies started turning their attention to another global health issue knocking at the door—cancer.

Chapter 14

A NEW CHALLENGE

In 2001, I got a call from the product leader for Glivec, a drug for a destructive and prevalent cancer called chronic myeloid leukemia (CML), made by the pharmaceutical company Novartis. The call had a profound impact on me. So much so that I remember—among the thousands of calls I've had since—that she called me at 5:30 in the evening on a dark winter day. The call was prompted by a recent announcement by the then CEO of Novartis, who declared that no patient in need of CML treatment should be left behind simply because of inability to pay or where they happen to live in the world. The September 11 terrorist attacks had resulted in a new wave of global cooperation and solidarity. PEPFAR, launched that same year, was an output of this new wave, and the CEO's comments partially were as well.

Novartis's question that night was not an easy one to answer: How do we get Glivec to people all over the world? Glivec had just been approved by the FDA in 2001 and it wasn't like any other cancer treatment. It was a game-changer. Glivec was the first in a new group of drugs known as targeted therapy, and much like ARVs did for HIV, it had the potential to turn CML from a deadly disease to a chronic one. They had heard about my work on HIV and about Axios and they wanted to see how we could help design a global program for Glivec. Novartis's CEO was a physician himself and was serious about the commitment not to leave patients behind.

When I hung up, I thought, "Wow, this is happening. I wasn't so crazy after all. The private sector is taking the lead." At a time when the world wasn't even thinking about cancer, the private sector, driven mostly by market forces, and to some extent, the global solidarity dynamics of the time, was already thinking of the next step. I know many of you may be thinking, "Of course, they just wanted to make money." And you wouldn't be wrong. I do think their main driver was to safeguard their primary markets in rich countries. They also wanted to avoid a situation similar to what we experienced with ARVs where drugs were donated or priced at nonprofit prices. While those solutions helped many AIDS patients, they were not financially sustainable for companies. Financial incentives are responsible for many of the world's greatest medical treatments. Once companies no longer saw a financial incentive to continue, generics took over and the pipeline for needed HIV medicines dried up.

The Glivec story is an extraordinary one, but before I tell you more, I want to acknowledge an important point. I've worked with pharmaceutical companies since the early '90s and I know they aren't perfect. They have substantial issues that need to be addressed. In fact, Axios was created to confront a problem pharmaceutical companies are largely responsible for: the high cost of medications. I've told you about several instances when they were slow to react and hesitant to adopt a new way of thinking about access to treatment, much like the public sector. The difference is that financial incentives pushed them beyond their comfort zone faster. That's why I think it's necessary for the healthcare system to be more accepting of solutions that bring multiple parties to the table. Not because private is good and public is bad. Not because Axios clients are private pharmaceutical companies, but because there are urgent gaps in the healthcare system that need to be addressed as quickly as possible, and I believe that together we'll get there faster. With the Viramune Donation Program (VDP), for example, NGOs and private clinics were able to start the program and begin serving patients faster than governments. Yet it wasn't until governments also began implementing VDP that the program was able to grow to scale and provide Viramune to a larger, broader group of pregnant women. The private and public sectors have complementary roles to play. When our healthcare system welcomes all sides—public, private, and everyone in between—we can save more lives.

Over the next few chapters, I will share several stories from treatment access programs conducted by Axios with financial support from pharmaceutical companies. The point of these stories is not to promote Axios or to celebrate these companies. The point is to illustrate a different, more collaborative way of delivering healthcare—a way that is not exclusively centered on the hospital and invites several parties to support patients in a more holistic way. This more collaborative approach to healthcare delivery is one I've seen work better for patients many times over, and that's why I want to share it with you. The Glivec International Patient Assistance Program, or GIPAP, is an excellent example.

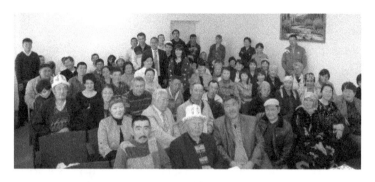

A group of patients from Kyrgyzstan enrolled in GIPAP came together during a site visit to share their experiences and give their feedback on the access program.

GIPAP, which became the first cancer access program in the world, was built on learnings from VDP. We put in place specific criteria that doctors and organizations—public and private—had to meet in order to be able to enroll in the program as Glivec providers. The program was implemented in both developed and developing countries. Axios managed the bulk of the low-income countries, and a US-based nonprofit, the Max Foundation, ran the programs in more developed countries. Axios was in charge of identifying, assessing, and recommending institutions for GIPAP and ensuring that drugs were properly stored and tracked by the GIPAP institution/physician and delivered to the patient. The Max Foundation was responsible for providing support and information to patients, guiding physicians and patients through the GIPAP application process, and reviewing and verifying patient eligibility.

One big difference from VDP was that sustainability was a primary objective of GIPAP. Glivec had turned cancer into a chronic disease and Novartis knew that once a patient received Glivec, they may need to be on treatment for many years. Donation programs are never sustainable. It's not financially possible to provide more and more patients with free medicine every year for eternity. At some point, the money runs out or takes away from other critical health needs.

Novartis wanted to set up this program in a way that would allow it to run for a long time, at least until their patent ran out and a generic version of Glivec became available. We worked with them to assess a range of different scenarios. Despite the fact that dual pricing (where drugs are priced differently for different countries) for HIV/AIDS drugs had become a fairly acceptable practice by the early 2000s, Novartis was not yet interested in dual pricing for GIPAP. They wanted to maintain one price around the world for many of the same reasons we heard from companies during DAI. By 2009, they eventually came around to the idea for more developed nations.

In the meantime, the decision was made to provide the drug for free to those who could not afford it in low-income countries. In middle-income countries, if patients weren't covered by their insurance or the government, they could also receive the medication for free. Otherwise, they paid full price. As a whole, this model allowed wealthier patients to subsidize those who could not afford it, making the program more sustainable than a program that was fully donation-based. While the model had its challenges (more on that in the next chapter), it was the first time the idea of access sustainability entered the consideration set. Up until GIPAP, access was about short-term donations.

GIPAP came at a time of transition in global health. Cancer had started to show its heavy hand, but most low- and middle-income countries were primarily preoccupied with HIV/AIDS. The burden of cancer seemed insignificant compared to the millions dying of AIDS every year. But our friends in Tanzania and throughout the world told us a different story. The Director of Tanzania's Muhimbili Hospital told us now that AIDS patients were on ARVs and had mostly left the hospital, his wards were instead filling up with diabetes and cancer patients.

The cancer issue had escalated quickly. In a span of five years, cancer in the developing world went from an invisible issue to one of major concern. Rapid urbanization in low- and middle-income countries brought about pollution, changes in nutrition and physical activity, and contributed to the rapid rise of cancer incidence. Plus, as science progressed and the international community rallied around treatments, cancer became more visible.

Unsurprisingly, health systems were largely ill-prepared to deal with this new and rapidly growing challenge. Tests weren't available. Doctors weren't trained. Hospitals were quickly over-whelmed. By 2007, cancer was killing more people each year globally than AIDS, tuberculosis, and malaria combined, and more than 70 percent of the global cancer burden was found in low- and middle-income countries. Yet when GIPAP first began enrolling patients, few paid it much attention.

Given the severity of the issue, as Axios, we felt that we had a responsibility to bring attention to it. We were much more implementation-minded, but we also knew the power of policy. In HIV, an aligned scientific community combined with a com-pelling reason for action and a clear solution had successfully moved policymakers, and cancer needed much of the same. Policy shaping isn't easy—but it's a critical piece of the public health puzzle. Without it, long-term change and improvement are unlikely. When proper policies are in place, investment and funding followed—from the public and private sectors alike.

We tried as much as possible to replicate the kind of advocacy that we saw worked with HIV. To do that, we worked to create forums that raised awareness of not only the magnitude of the issue but also the solutions already available to address it. Through GIPAP, we built connections with important cancer stakeholders. Using those connections, Anne, who was Axios's Chief Technical Officer, spearheaded the development of an informal working group on cancer treatment in developing countries called CANTREAT International. The group, composed of experts from many leading global cancer organizations working in an individual capacity to develop new models for cancer care and treatment, was instrumental in putting cancer on the public health agenda.

In an editorial published in the *Annals of Oncology* in 2010, CANTREAT encouraged the public health community to remember the HIV/AIDS experience.[21] We called for multi-sector collaboration to help mobilize and increase cancer prevention solutions around the world. We also advocated for access to treatment, which we knew had greatly reduced illness and death during the HIV/AIDS pandemic and resulted in countless other improvements, from increasing patient interest in diagnosis and prevention to building healthcare provider knowledge and facilitating policy change. Through CANTREAT, our goal was to present one combined scientific voice with a clear path forward. That same year, we published a consen-

---

21 CanTreat International, "Scaling Up Cancer Diagnosis and Treatment in Developing Countries: What Can We Learn from the HIV/AIDS Epidemic?" *Annals of Oncology* 21, no. 4 (April 1, 2010): 680–82, https://doi.org/10.1093/annonc/mdq055.

sus paper during the World Cancer Congress in the southern Chinese city of Shenzhen. The paper painted a dire picture of the incredible toll that cancer was playing in low- and middle-income countries and the critical interventions needed to stop that momentum.[22] Our paper was covered by many international media outlets.

Once the issue gained global attention, then governments, public health agencies, companies, and researchers began to take note. GIPAP began to gain momentum, too. Between 2001 and 2014, 63,000 patients were helped in 93 countries. Although the number of patients reached may not seem particularly high, remember that we are talking about a rare disease. It was only one treatment for one type of cancer, but it was a start, and it gave people hope that access to quality cancer medications in developing countries was possible. We also shouldn't forget the systemic improvements that resulted from the program and their impact on future generations of patients. According to an impact analysis of the program, GIPAP positively impacted service delivery, access to care, diagnostic capacity, and health workers' skills at institutions involved with the program. Improvements in the utilization of disease guidelines, patient tracking systems, and institutional operations were also reported. Plus, 65 percent of physicians involved in the study indicated that their institutions had undertaken initiatives to increase access to cancer treatment after implementing GIPAP.

These results speak to the power of treatment access: when a solution becomes available, the demand for that medicine

---

22 Felicia Knaul et al., "Access to Cancer Treatment in Low- and Middle-Income Countries: An Essential Part of Global Cancer Control," *A CanTreat Position Paper*, CanTreat International (2010), https://papers.ssrn.com/sol3/papers.cfm?abstract_id=2055441.

increases. Treatment creates more incentive to build the proper infrastructure to support the provision of treatment. From more treatment facilities to more skilled providers, these infrastructure improvements in turn bring more patients into the fold. A stronger infrastructure also means more capacity for conducting disease awareness, which in turn drives up diagnosis rates and further increases the pool of patients receiving the treatment they need.

What I just described is a bottom-up, market-driven method of building infrastructure focused on stimulating the environment and local capacity. It's a method often used by private companies, while the public sector tends to prefer a top-down approach, blocking the development of local healthcare initiatives in the process, as we said in the previous chapter. For example, say there is a need for a hospital in a city. The top-down approach says, "I am putting a hospital here." The bottom-up approach says, "There is a need for a hospital and we should encourage someone to build and run it." Governments can put significant hurdles in place that can discourage a bottom-up approach. We saw that in Vietnam with DAI, in Tanzania with the traditional birth attendants, and in many other countries we operated in. For just that reason, Axios's access programs weren't always easy to get off the ground. They were seen as innovative or as outliers, depending on who we talked to. But in the end, once we persevered and overcame the obstacles put in our way, they made a difference with patients.

As cancer took an ever-increasing toll in poorer countries and pharmaceutical company pipelines began to fill with cancer medications, we felt it was time to reach out to companies to ask if they were interested in helping. Women's cancers was one area Axios and the CANTREAT experts felt required specific attention. That's why we were happy to hear from AstraZeneca, the manufacturer of several breast cancer drugs. They were eager to start an initiative in Africa and asked us to support them in a capacity-building and treatment access project in Tikur Anbessa Hospital in Addis Ababa, Ethiopia, the reference hospital in the country.

Worldwide, breast cancer is the most diagnosed cancer and the leading cause of cancer death in women. Currently, just under half of all new cases and most deaths occur in the developing world. Diagnostic and treatment services are limited, and most patients are first seen when the disease is advanced. In sub-Saharan Africa, only 32 percent of women are still alive five years after diagnosis, compared with 81 percent in the US.

As we had done with HIV, our goal was to show that breast cancer treatment in Africa was feasible with the proper foundation. At the start of the project, there was a single oncologist for the whole country of 100 million people and only one radiotherapy unit in Ethiopia. There was no estrogen and progesterone hormone receptor test; no access to life-saving cancer drugs; and limited awareness of breast cancer among health workers and the public.

The project began with an assessment of needs at Tikur Anbessa Hospital. Together with hospital staff and the Ethiopian Cancer Association, Axios developed a plan for a six-year project to strengthen breast cancer management and treatment and to raise public disease awareness to improve diagnosis.

The plan included specific interventions to build hospital

capacity, like the installation of mammography and ultrasound equipment, training for doctors, pathologists, and lab technicians, and the implementation of patient management and follow-up systems. We also planned to improve the capacity of physicians in regional hospitals so they knew when to refer a patient for follow-up in a specialized hospital with more training in breast cancer diagnosis, like Tikur Anbessa. Once diagnosed, treatment was provided to patients free of charge.

We had learned from Muhimbili and our experience with TBAs that we needed to look beyond the hospital too, and so that's what we did in Ethiopia. Support was provided to the Ethiopian Cancer Association to help build their capacity to raise disease awareness, educate patients, and fundraise. Just like HIV/AIDS, disease awareness and early diagnosis were major gaps. If a patient didn't know what breast cancer was, and if, how, and where it could be treated, it was unlikely that they would come into the hospital until it was too late. And that's exactly what was happening. At first, we literally had to go out and find patients, but over time, that changed.

I remember stories from countless women who became disease advocates after participating in the project. During one of my visits to Ethiopia, I met Aida. Aida's cancer crossed the skin and became apparent. She told me that at first, people thought she was bewitched. She was taken to the shaman, then to a traditional healer, and finally to the regional hospital after everything else failed. Unfortunately, Aida was past the stage where surgical removal could help. Only radiotherapy, chemotherapy, and palliative treatments were possible. Regional hospitals could not deliver cancer treatment, so they sent her to Tikur Anbessa. Our referral system was working!

There was also Senait. After her treatment, she began working at a Family Guidance Clinic where she promoted breast self-examinations, pap smears, use of contraceptives, and as appropriate, referred women to the hospital for more specialized medical assistance.

And how can I forget Menbere? I remember her telling us that she knew many women in her community who had died of breast cancer because of stigma and discrimination. "In my culture, people don't want to talk about this disease," she said. She told us about a woman in her neighborhood who had breast cancer but chose to go to a traditional healer and take holy water and later died. After that and her own diagnosis, she made a point of telling anyone who would listen about what proper care and treatment looks like and the importance of early diagnosis.

As part of the project, we also worked with the government to develop clinical guidelines for breast cancer treatment and palliative care. As was the case in Tanzania, we had a great champion in Ethiopia—the then Minister of Health. During his time as Minister, from 2005–2012, he led a comprehensive reform of the country's health system. The transformation he led improved access to healthcare for millions of people. Under his leadership, Ethiopia invested in critical health infrastructure, expanded its health workforce, and developed innovative health financing mechanisms. When we first met with him before starting the project, I remember him telling me that cancer was not his priority. He had to focus on HIV and malaria and ensure that his people had access to essential medicines. But he also told me he was open to new initiatives like our project in Tikur Anbessa. Although he couldn't put Ministry resources behind the project, he was eager to be kept apprised of its progress. I understood his response. It was a practical one. He had to prioritize, but he was sufficiently forward-thinking to not block the innovation that we were proposing.

By late 2008, the number of patients screened, diagnosed, or treated at Tikur Anbessa increased tenfold. Using a multistakeholder approach that combined the government, a drug manufacturer, doctors, and patient organizations, we were able to build an infrastructure to diagnose and treat patients and to strengthen patient organizations and referral systems. The success of the program and the awareness created encouraged the Ministry of Health to take it to the next level. The country put in place a National Breast Cancer Plan that was included subsequently in a broader National Cancer Plan done in collaboration with WHO. Care and treatment guidelines and policies were developed in close collaboration with hospital staff, and a sustainability plan was developed to ensure the continuity of the project beyond the pilot. AstraZeneca also offered the country a discounted price for its breast cancer treatment.

Like GIPAP, the Ethiopia project catalyzed the development of an appropriate infrastructure to improve cancer management in the country for the long term. A lot more work would be needed to reach the infrastructure level of middle- or high-income countries, but the fundamental elements were now in place.

We had a model that we knew worked, but how could we scale these solutions to more countries and more patients? Axios's CTO, Anne, had written the following as part of an editorial in the *Annals of Oncology*:

The knowledge and experience exist today to take effective action and to make a significant difference to cancer outcomes in low- and middle-income countries (LMICs). Cancer control is a human right. The challenge is to apply that knowledge through a public health framework to maximize the benefits for as many as possible while keeping costs at a manageable level for poorer countries and donors alike. Pilot programs are good, but they are insufficient. We now need to go to scale with what we know to be cost-effective interventions. In order to implement what we know, on a large scale, much greater resources are needed. Professional organizations, multilateral organizations, advocates, activists, and governments of LMICs must come together to advocate for action against cancer and for the funding to do what we know is right. The longer we wait, the greater the challenges will be. The time for action on cancer in developing countries is now.[23]

I couldn't agree more. But the way forward wasn't so clear. While these early programs moved us forward incrementally, they also showed us cancer was a different beast.

Cancer treatments were significantly more expensive than primary care medicines, or even ARVs. Treatment was long-term, and that meant different implications on access and the health system and in how companies responded. There were also big gaps of time between what are called "blockbuster" treatments, or treatments that represent significant advancement from previously available treatments. Many new drugs were simply me-too products with small incremental improvements from already available medications. Modest improvements aren't likely to mobilize a global response.

---

23 CanTreat International, "Scaling Up Cancer Diagnosis."

Cancer also didn't attract the big funds like HIV did, or even the same level of advocacy. It was too fragmented. There were many kinds of cancers. Some were rare, while others wreaked havoc on a country. That meant a wide range of stakeholders and many different types of patient groups and advocates, each pushing for their own agenda. We can compare the situation with climate change. The climate change movement brings together a wide range of issues—energy, animal extinction, food sustainability, weather, etc. There's no clear problem or clear solution. As a result, despite significant urgency, we've made little progress, and the progress we have made is often reversed as political administrations change.

Politicians will not make decisions on complex problems. You have to break the problem into pieces and identify a clear and workable solution to each piece. Make it easy for them to digest. That's how we accomplished what we did with HIV. Despite the many treatment combinations, we had one treatment solution— ARVs—that prevented people from dying. We demonstrated that this treatment solution could be effectively used in Africa and had the entire scientific community speaking in one voice.

Which brings me to what I feel is the most important reason why cancer has never gotten the attention it deserves: there has never been one straightforward solution for people to get behind. We tried hard to create this through CANTREAT by rallying the global community behind access to cancer treatments, but the conditions weren't there to drive the momentum. With HIV, there was worldwide outrage and a global call for collaboration to lower the price of ARVs. There were many other issues beyond treatment, but homing in on the most blatant, visible issue allowed the public health community to respond in sync.

For cancer, however, the World Health Organization issued its first cancer resolution in 2005.[24] That resolution mostly drew attention to the issue, but said little about solutions. It wasn't until 2017—twelve years too late—that it published another resolution, this time emphasizing the urgency of solutions to improve accessibility and affordability of cancer care.[25]

With cancer, all we had was a clear problem, and a growing realization that the solution is one we'll have to find on our own. Thankfully, we had nearly two decades of learnings to guide our way.

24   World Health Organization, "WHA58.22: Cancer Prevention and Control," in *Fifty-Eighth World Health Assembly*, 92–7, May 25, 2005, https://apps.who.int/gb/ebwha/pdf_files/WHA58-REC1/english/A58_2005_REC1-en.pdf.

25   World Health Organization, "WHA70.12: Cancer Prevention and Control in the Context of an Integrated Approach," in *Seventieth World Health Assembly*, 22–6, May 31, 2017, https://apps.who.int/iris/bitstream/handle/10665/259673/A70_REC1-en.pdf?sequence=1&isAllowed=y.

Chapter 15

CAN WE REACH EVERYONE?

During my time working in HIV, I remember many moments where I felt frustrated with the lack of action, slow response, or unwillingness of my colleagues to step outside their comfort zone. But I don't remember many moments where I felt at a loss in terms of what to do next. I also don't remember feeling alone. Although we weren't always in agreement, there was an entire world banded together in outrage against HIV. With cancer, it was different.

No one was knocking on our door for answers. No activists pushing companies to do more. No conversations with governments eager for solutions. Only patients suffering.

The evolution of cancer and other noncommunicable diseases (NCD) and chronic diseases, like heart disease, stroke, and diabetes, seemed to come out of nowhere. The world had been so consumed by HIV for so long that we missed the clear warning signs. Driven primarily by four major risk factors—tobacco use, physical inactivity, alcohol use, and unhealthy diets—NCDs were quickly becoming responsible for the majority of deaths worldwide, with most of those deaths happening in low- and middle-income countries.

I remember a conversation I had with Anne, Axios's CTO that I mentioned earlier. We were in Zanzibar, Tanzania. It's a beautiful place, perfect for coming up with new ideas. Both of us had been deeply involved in HIV when companies were making huge donations and putting down incredible amounts of money knowing that they were getting nothing in return. What may they be willing to invest, and for how long, if we could make these access solutions worth their while financially? That question was the impetus for what became a huge shift—first at Axios and later across much of the access to healthcare industry.

We set out to find the answer.

By the early 2000s, the pharmaceutical industry was going through major shifts. In the '80s and '90s, bottom lines were largely driven by antibiotics, antihypertensives, and heart disease medicines. They were easy to sell, sold in huge volumes, and most governments covered their costs. Antibiotics and other primary care medicines made companies huge profits until generics took over. Eventually, when the HIV epidemic entered the scene, some companies also began to invest significantly in the development of antiretrovirals. But like primary care medicines, once more and more generic ARVs began appearing, the HIV research and development engine came to a grinding halt. Instead, companies began shifting their focus to specialized medicines for chronic and noncommunicable diseases, autoimmune diseases, and other specialized conditions. These medicines were more complicated to manufacture, which made the generic development process lengthier and more complex—positive news for companies. Demand for these medicines was also increasing, driven by rising rates of NCDs.

Despite the demand for specialized medications, companies found themselves in uncharted waters. First, while the demand was there, it wasn't even close to the massive quantities of primary care medicines they were used to selling. These medicines were for specialized conditions, and thankfully, there weren't millions of patients requiring cancer treatment in a country every year. Second, and most importantly, the complexity of the research that went into developing these medications made them quite costly. Recovering the higher cost of development from a smaller pool of patients implied that the price of medicines had to be significantly higher than other medicines on the market. Glivec (and basically all cancer medications that would come later) fell into this category. It was out of reach for most of the world's population. Governments—especially in low- and middle-income countries—also did not have the necessary budget to cover the cost of these medications in full or even partially, as they had done for primary care medicines. Companies were used to selling lower-cost primary care medicines in huge quantities directly to governments, who would, in turn, reimburse patients in full or partially for the cost of the medication. Specialized medicines completely changed that game, and companies were unprepared to handle it.

The issue started to become very clear during the management of GIPAP. Let me explain. With GIPAP, patients who were poor received Glivec as a donation. Patients who were able to pay paid full price for the medication, or were reimbursed or covered by insurance. Despite the legitimacy of the rationale behind that model, which enabled patients who were able to pay to subsidize those that couldn't, segmenting patients into only two tiers— rich versus poor—still left many behind. What about that huge middle class in the center? Those who were too rich to receive a donation but too poor to pay full price and had no other coverage? The middle class in developing countries, especially in middle-income countries, was growing exponentially, yet they were being left out of the access equation. This meant a huge group of patients who could be getting treatment that weren't.

An Illustration of Why Donation Programs Don't Solve All Treatment-Access Issues for Higher-Cost Medications in Low- and Middle-Income Countries

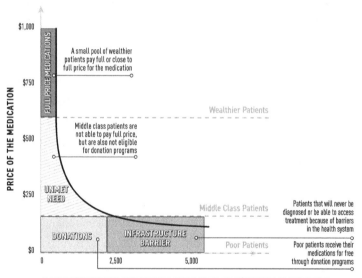

OF PATIENTS THAT CAN PAY FOR MEDICATION AT DIFFERENT PRICE POINTS

With traditional access approaches (like donation programs), the largest pool of patients, which tend to be those in the middle class, are not able to access treatment. Instead, creative access strategies make it possible for more patients to access treatment by enabling people who can pay more to subsidize people that can pay less.

It also meant a significant revenue source for companies was not being tapped. Tapping into this revenue source isn't just significant because it would make companies more money. It would also make the access solution more sustainable—in this case, GIPAP. What I mean is that if companies are making the necessary profits to continue supporting such programs and offering donations to patients that need it, the program will last longer and support more patients.

Remember Brian, the consultant that helped me during DAI negotiations? I remember him telling me that companies will charge what the market can pay, and not what the drug actually costs. That sentiment led to the novel idea that perhaps there was another way to charge for medications. Instead of one consistent price, or different prices for different countries, what about charging based on what a patient can afford? If you have more, you pay more; if you have less, you pay less. If you have ever been to a market in a poorer country, you are probably pretty familiar with this concept. If you look like an expat, you'll be charged more. If you are local, you'll be charged less. But in healthcare, it was entirely new territory to think about medication costs in this way. Until that point, medicine, like every other product, had a price. You could either afford it or not.

From the start, our mission at Axios was to increase access to treatment for all kinds of patients for the long term. Nothing had changed. We were just working with different variables in a different context. We were still very much driven by our mission, but we knew that we had to tap into companies' desire for profit if we wanted to achieve sustainable access for patients. We couldn't wait for governments to act. We had to move with the partners that had the most skin in the game and were most willing to move fast.

We started to explore solutions that would work for both patients and for pharmaceutical companies. The pharmaceutical industry has been the big bad wolf for a long time, and so it's not surprising that the idea of helping them make money (or not lose any, at least) in order to help more patients is an unpopular approach in the public health world. But I didn't get into public health to be popular. I got into this to help people, and I really thought this could work.

We weren't 100 percent sure where to start, so we began with a few assumptions.

We knew these treatments were expensive, and that getting pharmaceutical companies to bring down their prices would take years or wouldn't happen at all. And even if they did lower their prices, how low could they go? Many of these medicines were over US $3,000 a month. Even if you lowered it by 75 percent, you'd still have a huge part of the population that wouldn't be able to afford it. Plus, if you already have some patients paying the full amount, why do you want them to pay less? We also knew that while companies were no longer willing to donate their medicines for years and years, they may still be willing to make a contribution to the total cost of the medication—if we could make it worth their while. Plus, it was clear that governments in poorer countries were unlikely to be able to cover any significant portion of the cost of these medicines for their population. This meant the burden of paying for these drugs would largely fall on the patient.

To ultimately make these access solutions commercially sustainable, we had to create a balance across what the wealthy, middle-class, and poor were paying for treatment so that on average, across all patients, companies at least broke even and the largest number of patients were reached. Such a model would require each patient to pay a different amount for the drug based on their ability to pay, and for companies to cover the remainder.

The next obvious question was how do we know who pays what?

I reached out to my friend Joel (remember my colleague and friend from Rwanda?) to see if he could help. He had become a professor of public health at the University of Rouen in France, and after I joined Axios, we continued to collaborate on some research and analysis projects. He introduced me to Etienne, an epidemiologist who would later become a professor at Paris University. He is a wizard in statistics and math and helped us construct what we call the affordability model. The model used macroeconomic indicators to estimate the percentage of patients in a given country that could pay certain amounts for a given medication. Say a medicine cost US $5,000 per month. The affordability model was able to estimate how many patients could afford the medication at that cost and at multiple cost points below it. The purpose of the model wasn't to figure out the price of the medication. It was to understand, on average, how best to segment the population based on how much patients in that country were able to afford—and in turn help reach the greatest number of patients.

Novartis was the first company we approached with this idea. They were beginning to get increasingly worried about the huge number of donations under GIPAP and the very small number of patients paying full price for Glivec. If the trend continued in that direction, it wouldn't be long until they could no longer keep the program running.

Conceptually, they liked the idea of different patients paying different portions of the cost of treatment, with Novartis covering the rest. But they wanted to better understand how we would determine what an individual patient could pay. For example, the affordability model told us that 100 people could pay US $5000 a month and that 200 people could pay US $2,500, but it didn't tell us how we would determine which patient paid US $5,000 and which paid US $2,500.

It's helpful to be able to segment the population's ability to pay on a curve, but we wanted more than a theory. We wanted (and needed) something actionable that could be directly used to improve access to treatment. To achieve that, we needed a tool to assess an individual's ability to pay and one that would be sensitive enough to detect small differences in affordability in the real world. In other words, differences between the very rich and rich, the very poor and moderately poor. This level of segmentation is what would make the difference between a sustainable and a non-sustainable access model.

My colleagues at Axios began to look at tools that already existed to assess ability to pay. There were plenty out there, but none did exactly what we needed. Banks, for example, used these tools often when determining loan amounts, but it was in the best interest of the loan seeker to show that they were actually wealthier than they were or at least to show their wealth to get the loan. Charities had their own tools as well, but they only segmented the poor from the not poor. We ended up combining all of these tools, pulling their indicators, and creating our own tool to fit our needs. The tool we developed and validated in 2006 is what we call the Patient Financial Eligibility Tool, or PFET.

PFET is used to assess how much help a patient needs to cover the cost of treatment (based on their individual financial situation). It's the only patient assessment tool that takes into consideration not just income, but also assets and standard of living. Since we were mostly working in countries where informal economies prevailed, this kind of triangulation was important.

This is how it worked. Patients would participate in a financial assessment that asked them a series of questions—from more obvious questions like how much they make per month, to questions to better assess wealth levels, like the type of floor they have in their home, how many televisions or cars they have, how much they pay for school tuition, etc. These questions are customized per country. The patient's responses are then used to create a treatment plan that details how many boxes of their prescribed medication a patient will need to pay for and how many they will receive for free (with the cost covered by the pharmaceutical company that makes the product or sometimes other parties, like charities). The treatment plan was based on their entire course of treatment. This helped ensure that patients wouldn't need to drop out of the program because they ran out of money and could instead get the maximum benefit from their prescribed treatment.

You may be wondering why a company like Novartis was willing to accept patients not paying for their full course of treatment. Well, the shared payment approach I've described here allowed companies to keep the price of their medications the same. A patient pays the same for her box of medication as she would if she was paying full price, but the main difference is that she is paying for fewer boxes and still receiving her full course of treatment. This solution helped minimize pharmaceutical companies' drug diversion fears and created the potential for financial return, or enabled them to break even in markets where they were previously making zero or losing money.

The affordability model and PFET formed the core of what we termed "Creative Access Strategies," or CAS. It wasn't just a new model for access. It was an entirely new mindset based on sharing the cost of treatment. All of us at Axios felt that we had a very powerful model in our hands that could reverse the growing treatment access gap for specialty medicines in the developing world. We were eager to use it.

We continued our discussions with Novartis, and while they saw the value of this new model, they asked for exclusivity. Meaning that they wanted Axios to utilize the CAS model only with them. It's something we couldn't offer under our mandate to help patients.

With GIPAP under their belts, Novartis's understanding of access to treatment strategies was more advanced. Yet when we started discussing CAS with other companies, we hit a road-block. I felt like I was back in my DAI days. They knew they had to do something different, but found excuse after excuse not to pull the trigger. In this respect, they were similar to governments. Changing mindsets is never easy, but at least with the private sector, the promise of financial returns is a carrot they can't resist.

We just needed one champion to give this new approach a try and show what was possible. We soon found that in Pfizer. They had recently released a new cancer medication called Sutent. I received a call from the head of Public Affairs, and they, like Novartis, wanted to make it accessible to patients all over the world. We introduced them to CAS and they asked countless validation questions. It was a whole new way of thinking about medication access, and it took time to get them to come around. I remember long, sometimes contentious meetings working through their questions. Ebru, who began at Axios as a business school intern after writing a case study on CAS for INSEAD business school, was integral to this process—spending hours exploring different ways to cut the data and show companies the real value of this new approach. It wasn't an easy road, but in the end, the process helped us advance the model significantly and eventually led to the launch of the Sutent Patient Assistance Program, or SPAP.

We launched SPAP in ten countries in every corner of the world: India, Nepal, China, Malaysia, South Africa, Morocco, Philippines, Thailand, Pakistan, and Indonesia. Until this point, Axios was accustomed to implementing donation programs, but CAS meant a much more significant list of unnecessary barriers we had to overcome. A Sutent patient in one country is no different than one in another. Yet because of the divided health system we live with, every country meant different regulatory hurdles. Some required Ministry of Health approval in order to implement the program, others put tough regulations around donated products or pointless hurdles around product registration. I am very thankful for my cousin Najib, who happened to be an international lawyer, whom I brought on board to help navigate these endless roadblocks.

Here is how SPAP worked. Prescribing physicians would discuss the availability of SPAP with the patients prescribed Sutent. If a patient was interested, they would be referred to Axios's program manager in that country, who would, in turn, conduct a financial assessment of each patient using PFET. Based on the results, patients were provided with the financial support they needed in order to cover the cost of their full course of treatment. For patients unable to pay anything at all, the program provided the product for free.

At the time, we thought offering the product for free to those who weren't able to pay anything at all was the right thing to do. Our goal from the start was to reach as many patients as possible. Everybody, if possible, but SPAP taught us that this was not feasible.

First, because it made it financially unsustainable for the company. This became clear quickly. There were too many patients receiving donations and too few paying enough to balance out the cost of full donations. Second, there were infrastructure limitations that made it impossible to reach everyone. Poor patients didn't have access to diagnosis, for example. That was the reality.

We weren't ready to give up. We tried hard to find ways to make it more sustainable. Tax breaks were a possibility, and we explored a range of other avenues, but the program eventually had to be shut down because it became too expensive for Pfizer to maintain.

It was a tough lesson to learn. Reaching everyone was not possible. But at least we minimized the gap. It was better than nothing. We had reached many patients that would otherwise have never had access to Sutent. And we gave doctors desperate for something to offer their patients an option.

I learned a lot from the experience with Pfizer and am grateful for their willingness to try something new and grateful to Novartis for kickstarting this shift in mindset via GIPAP. In the end, I learned the hard lesson that real access wasn't going to be about reaching everyone. It was actually about reaching more. About ensuring that whoever we reach gets proper and complete treatment. There would always be those patients that couldn't be diagnosed or those so poor that there was no financially sustainable way to provide them with long-term treatment. Reaching everyone is theoretically great, but practically impossible.

I remembered those long nights at the emergency room in Lebanon surrounded by dozens of wounded soldiers. I knew I couldn't save them all. I saved many, but ultimately, I had to choose, with tears in my eyes. Theories are nice in mundane conversations, storybooks, or even science books, but not when patients' lives are on the line. In public health, when urgency is paramount, we must be willing to sacrifice utopia for necessity. I wasn't sure companies, countries, policymakers, doctors, and patients were ready for this reality.

Chapter 16

HEALTHCARE IN A FRAGMENTED WORLD

The idea of making treatment more financially accessible by asking patients to pay what they can afford and companies and other players to cover the rest was revolutionary. Until this day, I struggle to write that sentence. It sounds wildly boastful. But it's important to recognize. Not because Axios or I should be celebrated for it, but because it shows a key theme that I have been trying to illustrate in this book. What we called CAS was not just a new shiny toy. It had the potential to completely change how we think about how healthcare is paid for. Yet like the countless examples I've illustrated for you already, the expansion of CAS suffered as a result of our inflexible health system.

In our early days of trying to implement a shared payment model like the one used in SPAP, few companies were willing to give it a try. When we did have the opportunity to implement it, doctors complained that patients were asking why they were paying different amounts than their neighbors. Patients didn't want to undergo a financial assessment. Governments were upset that implementation was happening beyond their direct control.

It was frustrating to know we had something in our hands that could change the reality of so many sick people around the world, but the barriers put in our way seemed almost impossible to circumvent.

Then, the global financial crisis hit from 2008 to 2012. For Axios, we lost many of our major clients, and several others significantly scaled down their operations. But looking back, it was also a blessing. Let me explain.

The fifteen years that followed the end of the Cold War in 1991 were ones of relative peace and prosperity. Globalization and collaboration drove public health actions. Large global players like WHO, UN, PEPFAR, and Global Fund were seen as the main drivers of global health—swooping in to support low- and middle-income countries with massive aid packages, mostly in the form of treatment donations and large-scale infrastructure projects. HIV was still a big issue for many of these countries, but the availability of treatment had shifted significantly with the introduction of PEPFAR and Global Fund.

All of that came to a screeching halt in 2008 with the subprime crisis in the United States and the crippling effect of the global financial crisis that followed it. During the global financial crisis, a downturn in the US housing market was a catalyst for a financial crisis that spread from the United States to the rest of the world.

Foreign banks were active participants in the US housing market. US banks also had substantial operations in other countries. These interconnections provided a channel for the problems in the US housing market to spill over to financial systems and economies in other countries. Financial stresses peaked further following the failure of the US financial firm Lehman Brothers in September 2008. Together with the failure (or near failure) of several other financial firms around that time, global markets panicked. Investors pulled their money out of banks and investment funds. Banks incurred large losses and relied on government support to avoid bankruptcy. Businesses stopped investing and household spending dropped. Millions of people lost their jobs as major economies experienced their deepest recessions since the Great Depression in the 1930s.

In a nutshell, the 2008 financial crisis was devastating to the world economy. Yet without the financial industry's collaborative response, things could have been much worse. How much worse is something economists still argue over. It is tough to calculate the costs of bank bailouts, lost economic growth, and spiking public debt. But the biggest cost of the crisis might not be economic, but political and social: the populist wave that has swept over the world in the last decade, upending political systems, empowering extremists, proliferating inequality, and making governance more difficult. From Donald Trump in the United States to Jair Bolsonaro in Brazil, Victor Orban in Hungary and far-right candidate Marine Le Pen in France, the effects of the financial crisis are still very much alive today. We feel them every day in our increasingly nationalist politics and economies, and in the strengthening of non-democratic, totalitarian regimes such as those in China, Russia, and Turkey.

It's important to note that this response is nothing new. The world did something similar after the Great Depression. As the depression deepened, it had far-reaching political consequences. One response to the Depression was fascist and military dictators who promised to maintain order and restore economies. Instead, these power-hungry leaders refused to collaborate for the greater good—eventually leading to World War II. When resources are scarce, you want to keep them for yourself, not share them with the rest of the world. From nations to individuals—the financial crisis prompted the entire world to turn inward. Gone were the days of collaboration.

Yet there were two major differences between the Global Financial Crisis of 2008 and the Great Depression: the internet and globalization.

The internet and social media allowed us to see what the whole world was like without ever getting on a plane. It allowed us to continuously compare ourselves and what we had or didn't have with our neighbors—the ones next door and the ones across the world. On January 9, 2007, the iPhone put the world at our fingertips, and with it came an ever-increasing awareness of the world's haves and have-nots.

On one hand, we had governments preaching nationalistic views. We have to protect our own people. Stay within our borders. Do things our way. That's what they told us. But on the other hand, the forces of the information age were creating a common reality. We were all keenly aware of who had what. For those that didn't have it, it begged the question, why not me?

Meanwhile, the information age was also making a lot of people rich. Around 2010 or so, as countries and many critical industries struggled to recover from the Global Financial Crisis, the technology industry was beginning what is now a more than decade-long boom. That's partly because the tech industry was well insulated from the financial meltdown's real estate–focused epicenter. And Silicon Valley had already experienced its own financial bust in the early 2000s. Cash had flooded in from investors attracted by low interest rates set by central banks trying to stoke a broader recovery—with big payoffs.

Politically we were nationalists, but economically we were globalists. While the poor were told to be nationalistic, the rich had the world as their playground. Take the Panama Papers for instance. The Panama Papers were an unprecedented leak of 11.5 million files starting in 2016 from the database of the world's fourth-biggest offshore law firm, Mossack Fonseca. The documents showed the many ways the rich, including twelve national leaders and 143 politicians, were exploiting secretive offshore tax-havens.

As a result of all these factors, the gap between the rich and the poor became more obvious, further fueling dissatisfaction and dissent within and across countries, and prompting crises around the world.

This dichotomy also began to shift the notion of borders. A wealthy family in Tennessee in the United States had much more in common with a wealthy family in China or India than their neighbors down the street who were barely scraping by with an hourly job at McDonald's or no job at all. Our economic standing began to define us better than the country we were born in, the language we spoke, or even our religion. If we were all so different inside one country, what is the purpose of the border that divides us from neighboring countries?

In Yuval Levin's book, *The Fractured Republic*, he argues that we have moved to an age of decentralization where we've replaced attachment to large established institutions like governments with support for more flexible structures like our local communities.[26] I couldn't agree more. While the availability of the internet and social media bolstered our interconnectedness, it also created increasing levels of fragmentation in society far beyond our national borders. Today, we identify most closely with people who have similar interests to us or believe in the same causes. The result is a deeply divided society often uninterested in supporting the people that fall outside our immediate circle of comfort. That goes for individuals and governments alike.

I know I've painted a grim picture of the world at this time. But from my perspective, it's an accurate one. Both developed and developing countries were affected. No one was spared. With profits dropping in wealthier countries due to the crisis, companies of all kinds, including pharmaceutical companies, started to think about low- and middle-income countries as a potential complementary revenue source. That meant more attention and more investment in countries where there existed the greatest healthcare needs. At the same time, the tension between the haves and have-nots prompted a new momentum for interventions to minimize this double standard. These shifts would take time to come to fruition, but this is why I told you the Global Economic Crisis was both a curse and a blessing for Axios and for the patients we hoped to support.

---

26 Yuval Levin, *The Fractured Republic: Renewing America's Social Contract in the Age of Individualism* (New York: Basic Books, 2016).

For the bulk of the 20th century, the middle-class consumers of North America and Europe have been the source of demand, while low- and middle-income countries in Asia, Africa, and Latin America have been the source of supply. However, following the economic crisis, American and European households began saving in an effort to rebuild lost wealth, with a significant impact on consumption. How could the world economy fill this void in global demand? All eyes turned their attention to emerging markets, primarily Asia, where a growing middle class was preparing to become the next global consumers.

By combining household survey data with growth projections for 145 countries, economists projected that Asia accounted for less than one-quarter of the world's middle class in 2010, but that share was estimated to more than double in the next ten or more years—accounting for over 40 percent of global middle-class consumption.[27] This pattern could be seen in many higher-end developing countries at the time, but it was most obvious across Asia.

A growing middle class indicated more financial prosperity for many households, which translated to more disposable incomes to spend on healthcare, food, and other items. On one hand, this resulted in populations in these countries living longer. On the other hand, as fast food brands started popping up all over Asia, so did health conditions like obesity, diabetes, and high cholesterol. Both factors contributed to higher rates of noncommunicable and chronic diseases that are more likely to strike at older ages or in unhealthy individuals. This meant demand for specialized medicines to prevent or treat these

27   Homi Kharas, "The Emerging Middle Class in Developing Countries," *OECD Development Centre Working Papers*, no. 285 (January 2010), https://doi.org/10.1787/5kmmp8lncrns-en.

diseases was skyrocketing, but the funds to pay for it all were nowhere to be found.

Governments found themselves in quite a conundrum. They were used to reimbursing the cost of primary care drugs for their populations, meaning that many of their citizens received these medicines for a low cost or for free. But now they were faced with an entirely different reality altogether. They needed to cover more people with more expensive, specialized medications. Combine that with tightening budgets still reeling from the effects of the Global Economic Crisis, and governments were at a loss for how to pay for it all.

You may be wondering where was the UN and WHO in all of this? It's been a while since I mentioned them, and there's a reason for that. As countries became more nationalistic, they became less interested in multilateralism. They didn't want to give authority to the UN. They wanted to keep it for themselves. Funding streams also changed with a much higher percentage going to PEPFAR and Global Fund. As a result, the relevance of WHO and the UN went down significantly from the HIV days. Despite calls for change, they struggled to adapt to the changing world. They failed to understand that healthcare response goes beyond a medical response and multisectoral relationships are needed to address diseases on a global scale. HIV showed us that so clearly. But their dogmatic, rigid point of view held them back. As a result, the organizations assumed a largely normative role focused on developing guidelines and recommendations, despite the incredible need for a centralized healthcare body to shape policy and manage a global public health response. It also didn't help that in the internet age, normative institutions became largely irrelevant. What's the point of having country-level WHO guidelines that take years to create, when I can find the already approved, used, and validated guidelines from the US Food and Drug Administration or the European Medicines Agency in two clicks through a Google search?

One of the UN's and WHO's well-intentioned but out-of-touch interventions was Universal Healthcare (UHC). In 2005, the World Health Assembly issued a call on member states for UHC, with an aim to achieve affordable and accessible medical care for all citizens. It didn't get much traction until 2015, when all 169 UN member states adopted the Sustainable Development Goals (SDG)—a universal call to action to end poverty, protect the planet and improve the lives and prospects of the world's population by 2030. Achieving UHC is one of the SDG targets. WHO defines UHC as follows: "universal health coverage means that all people have access to the health services they need, when and where they need them, without financial hardship, including financial risk protection, access to quality essential health-care services, and access to safe, effective, quality and affordable essential medicines and vaccines for all."

The theory of UHC believes that "protecting people from the financial consequences of paying for health services out of their own pockets reduces the risk that people will be pushed into poverty because unexpected illness requires them to use up their life savings, sell assets, or borrow—destroying their futures and often those of their children." WHO states that 100 million people are driven into poverty each year through out-of-pocket health spending.[28]

28 World Health Organization, "Universal Health Coverage," accessed September 21, 2022, https://www.who. int/health-topics/universal-health-coverage#tab=tab_1.

Sounds great, I know. I think so too. In theory, at least. I have one question though: how are countries, especially poor ones, going to pay for it?

WHO suggests that efforts like pooling funds from compulsory funding sources (such as government tax revenues) can help. But there are limitations to that. A review of UHC programs around the world published in 2012 identified five factors for the success of UHC: the strength of organized labor and left-wing parties, adequate economic resources, absence of societal divisions, weakness of institutions that might oppose it (that includes, unsurprisingly, private insurance), and what's described as "windows of opportunity," with political leadership as the main one.[29]

If we compare what we know about the world now—divided, increasingly right-leaning—against that success criteria, it's no surprise that UHC hasn't delivered as much as we hoped.

Nevertheless, following the UN's call to action, many governments in low- and middle-income countries began to pursue UHC. Governments tried several UHC models with different delivery mechanisms and financial arrangements. Some were more successful than others, but none have yet managed to meet the end goal of enabling all people "access to the health services they need, when and where they need them."

On paper, UHC made governments look great. But in reality, UHC only covered basic medicines, not the specialty medicines needed to address the growing noncommunicable and chronic

---

29 Martin McKee et al., "Universal Health Coverage: A Quest for All Countries but Under Threat in Some," *Value in Health* 16, no. 1 (November 19, 2012): S39–S45, https://doi.org/10.1016/j.jval.2012.10.001.

disease rates. Soon patients on their deathbeds asking why they couldn't receive the treatments they needed started making headlines. Patients were left behind to pay out-of-pocket for these specialized medicines, making them a commodity only for the rich. By leveling from the bottom, UHC essentially formalized double standards between the rich and the poor.

A government couldn't come out and say directly that patients weren't covered for specialty medications. Instead, they began placing blame. Thailand, which began a UHC program in 2002, put it on the companies: "We aren't reimbursing patients because companies aren't reducing their prices." Mexico and Brazil kept delaying reimbursement decisions, hoping that their financial situation would change in the future. It hasn't. In Brazil, injunctions linked to patients suing the government for denying treatment have become commonplace as an access tactic. Most low- and middle-income countries also started to put in place increasingly complicated regulatory requirements for new products that made securing regulatory approvals and achieving reimbursement for new specialty medicines nearly impossible. They could have instead been transparent about not being able to cover more complex treatments for everyone and invited other players to help. But that didn't happen.

While healthcare was busy making its system harder and more complex, other industries were making it easier. After the financial crisis, the financial, trade, and retail industries took deliberate decisions to adapt to changing geopolitical circumstances and societal needs. These changes ultimately helped them recover from one of the darkest financial downturns in history. Banks created a range of platforms that made it simpler for all types of people to bank online, send money to friends and family, own their own business, and process their own transactions. The World Trade Organization put in place bilateral free trade agreements. The global commerce industry, with players like Amazon, turned the entire world into one big shopping mall. With one click, we could purchase goods from around the world and they'd arrive at our homes in only a few days.

Yet, not surprisingly, healthcare refused to budge. Instead of minimizing barriers to care, governments put more local regulations in place that made it harder to collaborate, to bring quality medicines to new markets, and ultimately to give patients the quality care and treatment they deserved. Healthcare remained a closely guarded domestic issue refusing to evolve while diseases and health threats globalized. Changes in our geopolitical environment over the twenty-first century, in step with changing technology, have had profound implications on the future of human rights, international relations, and, you guessed it, healthcare. As technology and globalization create an increasingly interconnected world, we must ask ourselves whether these artificial government-led barriers have any real value or whether they are getting in the way of our progress.

I know what you are thinking. Why put it all on the governments? Aren't the companies the ones causing this issue by charging astronomical prices for their products? That was often the pushback we heard from hospitals and doctors. The reality is that even with drastic price reductions, they would never be enough to reach everyone. Remember the price volume curve? We are not talking about a US $10 bottle of aspirin. We are talking about multi-thousand-dollar specialized medications for chronic and other deadly diseases. Even if the cost was cut in half, from US $4,000 to US $2,000, there would still be a huge group of patients not able to pay.

In essence, while UHC did improve access to basic medical coverage, it is unrealistic and unsustainable for the majority of countries when it comes to more advanced and expensive medicines. It also created an expectation that the government would provide for their healthcare. That expectation is not inherently bad, but it is when we know that the government will never be able to single-handedly provide for their entire population. Those that can afford to pay for medicine should, helping to subsidize those who can't.

Despite the best intentions, UHC contributed to the double standards we've already talked so much about because it uses an overly idealistic all-or-none model. By trying to give everyone the basics, countries ran out of money and couldn't give more specialized treatments to the few patients who really needed them. Instead, only those wealthy enough to pay for advanced, often more effective treatments were able to access them. Others were stuck with older, often subpar treatments. People began to demand better solutions, prompting an opportunity for others to fill the gap that governments simply couldn't fill alone.

Yet if the answer wasn't price drops or UHC, what was the alternative?

Many of the options we see in richer countries require a lot of money. For example, France's healthcare system is funded by a population who is wealthy enough to contribute a large percentage of their paycheck to health services. The French system costs 11 percent of the country's GDP—that's equivalent to Thailand's entire GDP. The UK, with its National Health Service, spends 12.8 percent of its GDP on health, and still, the wealthy pay for supplemental private insurance to guarantee quick, high-standard care.

The access landscape was at a standstill. Rising disease rates were met with better, specialized medicines to address them, but they were too expensive for developing governments. No global entity to coordinate or fund a sustainable response. A short-sighted, nationalistic point of view. Disillusioned patients with little disposable income being asked to pay out-of-pocket for life-saving medications. The world was putting everything on the patients' shoulders, contributing to an ever-growing division between the haves and the have-nots.

This was a really difficult time for Axios. While pharmaceutical companies were increasingly interested in developing countries, they weren't ready to put money on the table. Alternative access strategies were needed more than ever, but companies still felt their usual way of doing this would be sufficient. They also began to decentralize. Whereas Axios had a strong network of contacts within the HQ offices of many of these companies, we knew few in their country offices.

Internally, we were also divided. One half of the company was working on the remaining donation and infrastructure building programs from our early days. The other half was focused on new Creative Access Strategies. I waivered a lot between one or the other. It was clear that the days of huge pharmaceutical donations were gone, so that didn't seem like a viable path forward. But people like hanging on to what they have been doing. At the same time, I had no strong arguments for putting the whole company behind Creative Access Strategies at a point when there was limited interest from companies. I knew we couldn't keep doing both, but it took a while to get the courage to pull the trigger.

Axios was not doing well. We were losing money. I, along with other senior leaders in the company, had to defer part of our pay to keep the company afloat. It was becoming urgent to make a decision. I took one month off and fully disconnected from work. I went to Egypt to do my Divemaster training, and I volunteered as a diving guide on the diving school boat. I needed to disconnect, step back, and think. So much of my life was spent building up to this, and I was afraid to see it all crumble. I left UNAIDS because I strongly believed in the role of the private sector to drive change. Although the buy-in for alternative access strategies wasn't there yet, in the end, I trusted its immense potential to change the access landscape. My month underwater, totally disconnected, helped me see the big picture more clearly.

When I got back, I felt ready to make the move. I ultimately chose to shift the company's direction to focus solely on Creative Access Strategies, and with it came many internal shifts that required difficult decisions. We had to restructure the entire company—from our finances, to whom we hired, to our processes and procedures, and even to our clients. I'd be remiss not to mention Cliona, who joined Axios in 2009 as HR manager and stepped up far beyond her role to help me steer the ship back to profitable grounds. Her background was in HR, but she picked up finance, IT, and compliance seemingly overnight. I'm eternally grateful for her hard work and dedication in helping to redirect Axios into the company it is today.

It was a scary and draining time, but I believed in the long term we could accomplish so much more for patients through it. Patients around the world were taking on a level of burden they should never have had to do. That burden was growing by the minute along with the urgency for relief.

Chapter 17

SACRIFICING UTOPIA FOR NECESSITY: A LESSON IN SUSTAINABILITY

Somsak was a forty-nine-year-old Thai business owner. He was diagnosed with metastatic colon cancer in 2016, and his treatment was not covered by Thailand's Universal Healthcare program. As the family breadwinner, he decided that the amount he would have to pay for continuing his treatment was not worth the toll it would take on his family, including dipping into his children's education fund. "I decided to put my family's needs before my own. I could not be selfish and focus on myself." He ultimately chose to go without treatment. Somsak was a victim of the double standards that run so strong across our healthcare system.

Somsak's reality was one of many patients living in low- and middle-income countries. In the middle of all the geopolitical changes that resulted from the Global Financial Crisis, cancer had taken a back seat. It was a quiet epidemic. There was no worldwide outrage. But for those of us on the ground, the urgency was increasing.

The internet, social media, and the availability of digital technologies were diluting borders and bringing visibility to the world's double standards, along with escalated tensions. Pharmaceutical companies were investing in new, specialized medicines for chronic and noncommunicable diseases, but these medications came with a hefty price tag. There was huge demand for these specialized medications, but governments did not have the budget to cover their cost.

Pharmaceutical companies were eager to explore low- and middle-income countries as potential sources of revenue given decreasing spending power in the developed world, but they had no idea what to do in these markets. They may have donated medicines or worked with the government on huge tenders or bulk purchases for primary medicines, but those exercises didn't require a full understanding of how the landscape of that country worked. These interactions were largely transactional. Now companies found themselves having to figure out how to work closely with governments and sell to other stakeholders in countries they knew little about.

Early on, once they realized that government reimbursement wasn't going to happen and UHC had its limitations, companies began to offer what can best be described as bonus schemes to increase access to treatment in poorer countries. Patients were asked to buy a pre-set number of boxes of their medications to receive another pre-set number of boxes free—buy two, get one free, for example.

These schemes were short-sighted, and, I'd argue, unethical. Patients could perhaps make that initial purchase. Wealthier patients may even have been able to make a few more. But once the cash ran out, so did their treatment. You could say that patients should have the foresight to plan their long-term financial expenditures, but we all know that this is not how the world works. If you need treatment now, you are going to buy the box even if you know you may not have the money to buy the next round once the bonus boxes run out. With the best intentions, you hope you'll be able to figure it out and pull the money together in some way. But it's unlikely, frequently due to circumstances outside the patient's control. These bonus mechanisms started patients on a drug, only to take it away from them before they could fully benefit from it. The focus was on selling the box, not on supporting the patient and getting them healthier. It was a one-size-fits-all solution to a multi-layered problem.

This couldn't be the best that we could do. There had to be a better way.

We had learned a lot at Axios during our early pursuits of creative (or alternative) treatment access strategies. If I was to encapsulate every learning and realization we had, I'd say it came down to one critical observation: our goal was not just access to treatment. Our goal was *sustainable* access to treatment. In the case of chronic diseases or even noncommunicable diseases, a few boxes of medication wouldn't get you anywhere. It's not like aspirin where you take one pill and feel better. Feeling better required several cycles of treatment and sometimes lifelong treatment. Through our shared-payment programs, our hope was that giving the patient the ability to access treatment for as long as they needed it would not just improve their condition but also remove the incredible heavy financial and emotional burden that patients like Somsak had to deal with after being prescribed a treatment that cost five times their monthly wages.

I know "sustainability" is a boring, overused business buzzword, so let me define what I mean by it in this case. Sustainable healthcare access means 1) that a patient can pay for the cost of their treatment for however long they need it, and 2) that a pharmaceutical company can afford to support this access solution for the long term. This is commercial sustainability.

Given that by this time we were in large part supporting patients with chronic, long-term diseases, like cancer, the ability for an access solution to support a patient for as long as they needed to get the maximum benefit from their treatment was paramount.

At Axios, we began to dive deeper into our creative access strategy model to see how we could make it more sustainable.

With the Sutent Patient Assistance Program, we learned that the model of sharing the cost of treatment between the company and the patient was effective. Patients liked it. It gave them access to medication that they would otherwise never have been able to purchase. So did companies. It kept their price the same, allowed them to build their market in previously uncharted countries, and gave them a nice corporate social responsibility boost in the meantime. Physicians, for the most part, liked it too. Finally, they had an option for their patients. But unfortunately, with donations for patients who couldn't pay anything at all, it wasn't sustainable.

We knew that patients couldn't pay for the full cost of treatment on their own and they shouldn't have to. We also knew that most governments were not in a position to pay for it all either. While the precedent was that it was their responsibility to cover the cost of healthcare for their population, that precedent was established around medications that were one-twentieth of the cost of specialized medicines. Times had changed, and we couldn't keep doing the same thing. No one party could do it alone.

The Creative Access Strategies model allowed patients, companies, and potentially other parties to contribute to the total cost of treatment. We now knew that if we gave the product for free to anyone who couldn't afford it, the cost to the company would become too significant in contrast to what they were making from patients paying partially for treatment. What we had to figure out was how to make it sustainable by balancing out each party's contribution in a way that was affordable for the greatest number of patients, while making sure companies weren't losing money.

To do that, we had to first accept that there is a certain number of patients that we will not reach. Our early models applied incidence rates to the entire population and calculated that all those patients were potential candidates for treatment. But some patients would never even enter the healthcare system to be diagnosed and prescribed treatment simply because of other infrastructure barriers that exist. This is an issue, but one we wanted to tackle once we had addressed the glaring treatment access gap for the majority.

Second, we had to ensure that our tools to assess how much help a patient needed to pay for their treatment could pick up small differences in affordability. Those small nuances could have a big impact on the balance we were seeking.

Third, and this was a difficult one to accept, we had to implement a minimum payment unless supplementary funding (via charities or insurance for example) was made available. This meant that in order for a patient to enroll in the program, they had to purchase a preset minimum number of boxes. Each program would have a different minimum quantity based on where the break-even point was—the point where companies weren't losing money and the greatest number of patients were reached.

The idea of implementing a minimum was a tough pill to swallow. No pun intended. It went against the whole reason why we established this model in the first place. By asking patients to pay a minimum amount, it felt like we were contributing to the double standards we set out to diminish. But it was necessary. If we continued trying to find ways to prevent using a minimum to reach those not able to afford anything, we'd simply be losing time and holding back access from the many patients that could, in fact, afford some of it. We had to sacrifice utopia for necessity.

By 2013, limited success in low- and middle-income countries pushed some companies to finally start considering other routes. They had tried to use the same formula they followed in developed countries, and not surprisingly, it wasn't working. After several years of trying, governments were still hesitant or simply unable to reimburse expensive specialty medications. Bonus schemes where patients pay for a certain amount of boxes to get a certain amount free weren't panning out either, as most patients weren't able to keep paying for the full course of their treatment.

Out of necessity, some, like AstraZeneca and Novartis, started warming up to the idea of shared-payment access programs where multiple parties contribute to the cost of treatment. While it was still an uphill battle with many others, as was the case with countries during DAI, we forged ahead with the companies that were willing to step outside their comfort zone. We knew the others would come once these programs started to be successful.

Built on the learnings of some of our first-generation shared-payment access programs like Pfizer's SPAP, we focused this new wave of programs in Asia. As I mentioned earlier, Asia's middle class was booming, and among other developing economies at the time, they seemed to be best positioned for a program of this sort. Somsak was one of the patients we were able to help through one of our patient assistance programs in Thailand.

At this stage, the strategy for low- and middle-income markets was mostly being set out of pharmaceutical company headquarters in Europe or the United States. They were the ones that had given us the go-ahead to start in countries like Thailand and Malaysia. Country offices were more focused on implementation. HQ market access leads were eager to try something they had never done before. Their Asian country teams felt differently. Asian culture tends to be rather careful. They like to see how others do before they do it themselves. Once companies began to give more autonomy to Asia country offices to make decisions, growth in the region slowed down. Thankfully, Axios was already expanding to other regions of the world.

We started our Middle East operations out of Dubai in the United Arab Emirates in 2011 with the hire of our first program manager in the Middle East, Anas. For those of you that know Dubai for lavish shopping and exorbitant spending, the city might seem like a curious choice for a company whose mission was to expand access to healthcare. But Dubai was the regional hub for several pharmaceutical companies that served countries with a wide range of needs across the region. Second, there's a reason why Dubai is known worldwide for incredible feats of engineering like the world's tallest building, man-made canals in the middle of the desert, and ski slopes inside shopping malls. The UAE is fueled by innovation, and local market access leaders were always eager to try something new. They wanted to be the first, the largest, the best…and that mentality did wonders to drive uptake of shared-payment access programs. I should also mention that the UAE is home to 7.8 million foreign workers and their families. That's almost 90 percent of the population. Some of those immigrants are wealthy expats running the Middle East operations of some of the most profitable companies in the world, but the large majority are labor workers or service industry professionals with less purchasing power for high-cost, specialty medications. The remaining 10 percent of the population are Emirati, and their healthcare costs are fully covered by the government.

With the expat population growing in the UAE and rising rates of chronic and noncommunicable diseases requiring lifelong and/or costly specialty medications, healthcare companies and the government quickly acknowledged the urgent need for alternative access approaches. With the blessing of the Dubai Health Authority and the Ministry of Health, in 2012 we launched our first patient assistance program in the Middle East specifically for the UAE. It was called Musanda, a program Axios still manages today. The program was supported by Novartis and meant to increase access to several medications.

Patients prescribed these treatments were referred to the program by their prescribing physician. The patient then underwent a financial assessment by one of our Axios program managers to determine how much help they needed to pay for their full course of treatment. Novartis paid the remainder. Ever since the introduction of the minimum into our model, we were always on the hunt for other options that might help minimize the burden on patients who could not pay any of the cost. In the UAE, we realized we could tap into well-funded charities to support those patients. Our model in the country evolved into one where the cost of treatment was shared between the patient, the company, insurance companies, and local charities.

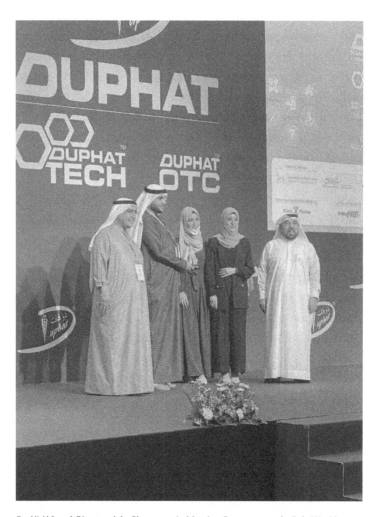

Dr. Ali Al Sayed, Director of the Pharmaceutical Services Department at the Dubai Health Authority, (first left), who is a key proponent of treatment accessibility in the UAE giving an award to the Axios Middle East and North Africa team at the DUPHAT 2022 conference.

Eventually, as we accumulated a critical mass of access programs in the country, the government also began to embrace our approach—thanks to champions like the head of pharmacy in the Dubai Health Authority. From our early days in the UAE, we worked closely with him to secure approvals for our programs. Yet as he saw more and more Axios access programs coming through his door, we began to talk about what it would mean to put in place an Emirate-wide access to medicines policy that was founded on the idea of shared payment. He had the foresight to see that a policy that spoke to the Emirate's commitment to access, including expats, and encouraged other players to come in to make it happen was a winning proposition for him and the country. Not only did it not cost him much more, but it also helped ensure that no patient was left behind.

In 2018, we helped the Dubai Health Authority develop its first access to medicines policy. As is always the case, once the policy was in place, the access to healthcare industry in Dubai grew significantly—soon more companies were interested in doing access programs, and we began to offer a broader range of patient services like adherence and nursing support. We had more competitors too, which only made us work harder. Entrepreneurship and competition drive innovation, which in turn drives better solutions for patients. I mentioned that before, and it applies to us (Axios) too. Our experience in the UAE is another great example of the importance of champions who are willing to think outside the box and bring in other players to make it work. It also speaks to the value of multi-sector, collaborative models to minimize the double standards we face in healthcare.

Our experience in Dubai prompted us to consider how we could implement similar models in nearby countries.

In Lebanon, for example, under the country's social security system, many treatments, including some of these specialized medicines for chronic diseases and NCDs were 80 percent covered by the government. Patients were expected to pay the remaining 20 percent per box. While there certainly were patients that could not pay the 20 percent, the biggest issue was that there were often delays in receiving the reimbursement check from the government for the 80 percent. This made it difficult to have enough cash on hand to cover the 20 percent on your next box. In this case, we began offering short-term financing to patients in the form of vouchers to cover their share of treatment. Patients would then repay the value of their voucher once funds became available. In other cases, where the patient could not afford the copay on their medication at all, we were able to offer vouchers to fully cover that cost, thanks to financial support from pharmaceutical companies and charities.

Our success in the Middle East was a game-changer. I must acknowledge the role of Anas and his leadership, who grew our Dubai office from one to over a hundred people in less than a decade. Today, we are serving thousands of patients in the region, and I am grateful to him for his tireless commitment to improving access. Anas was previously a nurse in the military and at first took a hefty pay cut to join Axios because he believed in our mission. I am sure that today, as Middle East and North Africa Senior Director, he sees that his decision paid off.

When companies began getting wind of the success in the Middle East, they began reaching out to see if we could replicate it in their own regions. Interest in Axios's alternative access programs picked up significantly. We hired Roshel, Axios's Senior Director of Global Consulting, who was charged with traveling the globe and answering the millions of questions that clients had for us. Can we trust the affordability model? How do we know what you are modeling will happen in real life? Will doctors refuse to accept a new solution? Is PFET accurate? The questions were endless. But we didn't mind them. It showed that there was interest and desire to try something new and different—and it's what we had been waiting for for a long time. I admit I did throw Roshel into the fire early on. Within her first month, I sent her to Thailand, Malaysia, and Singapore to work out a multi-country access platform with Takeda. I have a tendency to do that, but I knew she could do it. And she did. Soon, thanks to Roshel's foresight and tenacity, Takeda's access program, along with many others, expanded to Eastern Europe, Africa, and our friends in Asia came back too.

There was a mind shift happening in the access world, and I'd be remiss not to highlight the significance of that moment. Companies began to see that access is a multidimensional problem that requires multidimensional solutions, not one-size-fits-all ones. They saw the value of access sustainability and how it could be achieved and began looking at access as more than a corporate social responsibility endeavor. It had become a core part of their business. From the first day I stepped into a pharmaceutical company to try to convince companies to lower the prices of their ARVs and participate in DAI, I had been striving for this shift. It had taken almost twenty years, but it was finally happening. This shift won't solve our access problems overnight, and we still need many other players to come on board. But it's the start of an important movement toward a world where patients don't need to decide between feeding their families or taking their medication. I am incredibly proud of the role that Axios, and the many people and partners involved in our efforts, had in driving this shift.

When treatment is available and accessible, everything changes. Patients have more incentive to seek disease education and diagnosis because they know there is something they can do about it. Governments are more willing to invest in infrastructure improvements. Doctors and nurses are relieved of the burden of not being able to offer patients the care they need. I still remember vividly what it felt like to have nothing to offer Pascal in my early days as an infectious disease doctor. Week after week, I entered the exam room for his check-up, helpless and defeated. As his condition deteriorated, although I did the best I could, all I could offer him were a few pills to make him more comfortable. While I couldn't help Pascal as much as I would've liked, it gives me peace to know that I was able to help many others through our work at Axios.

Chapter 18

MORE THAN AFFORDABILITY: CLOSING THE GAP OUTSIDE THE HOSPITAL

Ironically, making treatment available and accessible to a point where a patient can stay on it for the long run has one somewhat counterproductive outcome—patients aren't good at staying on their treatment for the long run.

Over time, your average patient gets complacent with treatment. Once they start feeling better, they may stop taking it consistently, or at all. They forget to pick up their medications on time. They experience side effects that may not have been there early in their treatment. All of this requires a patient's doctor and nurse team to monitor their treatment carefully and closely. But when was the last time you got a call from your doctor or even your doctor's office to make sure you were staying on treatment or taking it as prescribed? It's been a while, if it ever happened, I am sure.

Doctor's offices are not set up for that kind of follow-up. Not only are they busy with an ever-growing patient load and paperwork, but the reality is that patient follow-up between appointments is not something that your everyday doctor's office sees as their responsibility. There's a historical reason for that.

The care of the sick began as a mostly religious endeavor. Eventually, holding areas for the sick were created, but little to no treatment was provided. These areas were a place for people to die, not a place to receive care. It wasn't until the seventh century that we began to see hospitals in the way we know them today. In fact, the first "modern-day" teaching hospital was founded by Abu Bakr al-Razi, a prolific physician and philosopher, in Bagdad, Iraq, in the ninth century. It is said that al-Razi chose the location of the hospital by hanging pieces of meat in various quarters of the city and finding the quarter in which the putrefaction of the meat was the slowest.

Early hospitals were built around the premise of having patients come to one place for care and treatment, versus the doctor walking for days to reach you at home. It was established as the center of care and hub of healthcare delivery. Hospitals were all about caring for the patient while inside their walls, but not when they leave. That's because early hospitals mostly treated very sick people or infectious diseases. Patients under the hospital's care were either quickly cured or died. While today we may have more sophisticated ways of picking the location of a new hospital that don't involve hanging a piece of meat, our vision of the hospital, or any healthcare clinic or medical office, remains the same.

Yet the world has radically changed since al-Razi's hospital. The size of our population has ballooned to 7.9 billion. We are living longer, eating unhealthy foods, and sitting at our desks for hours at a time—all factors contributing to a rise in diseases requiring lifelong, daily chronic medical treatment. Our hospitals and healthcare providers are overburdened and can no longer do the job alone. Add to it the growing risk of pandemics, and it's more than clear that the healthcare system needs to evolve to welcome other parties to complement traditional care providers. The COVID-19 pandemic is a perfect example of that.

Healthcare workers spent two years working around the clock to treat COVID-19 patients in overwhelmed hospitals. These hospitals were never set up to deal with this rapid influx of patients. Around the world, they rapidly reached full capacity, requiring patients to be treated in hallways, transported to other facilities miles away, or at times, not treated at all. It reminded me of the scenes we experienced at Muhimbili Hospital in Tanzania during the HIV/AIDS pandemic. As hospitals desperately tried to control the pandemic, did every other disease or condition requiring treatment go away? No, they didn't. Children didn't receive their recommended vaccinations. Chronic disease patients delayed their treatment for fear of going to the hospital and catching COVID-19, and critical surgeries were put off. Under these conditions, providers dealt, as best as they could, at least, with the mental devastation of losing patient after patient and the ongoing fear of infection. They were tired, overworked, and many quit. By 2030, there will be an estimated global shortfall of more than 10 million nurses, with the number of new nurses being outpaced by the number who are retiring, according to the World Health Organization's "State of the World's Nursing Report." Current levels of pandemic burnout will only exacerbate the staffing gap.

The incredible burden placed on providers and hospitals during the COVID-19 pandemic made headlines all over the world. Doctors were interviewed on live TV pleading for help and trying to draw attention to the issue, while terrifying scenes of patients struggling to breathe as they waited for ventilators played behind them. Despite the alarming headlines, this is not a new issue. It was just easier to hide it before a global pandemic hit us. Yet the healthcare sector continues to resist change. We continue to centralize care in one place and ignore the fact that much of a patient's care and treatment journey takes place once they leave the hospital.

If you think about the last time you were sick, did your journey end the second you walked out of the hospital or clinic? No. In fact, it was probably only starting. The real journey, the one that will impact whether you fully recover or get sick again, happens when you go home and have to make daily decisions about your care and treatment on your own.

This is particularly true for chronic diseases, which now make up a significant portion of the leading health conditions affecting the world, and where patient follow-up is particularly important. Adherence to long-term therapy for chronic illnesses in developed countries averages 50 percent. This means that, on average, patients take half of their treatments properly. As a result, they are unlikely to achieve optimal medical outcomes. In low- and middle-income countries, the rates are even lower.

Poor adherence to long-term therapies severely compromises the effectiveness of treatment, making this a critical issue in population health. It also increases overall healthcare costs by contributing to risk factors that will require further medical intervention.

In 2003, the World Health Organization put forth a multidimensional model that moved away from "blaming" patients or healthcare providers and instead proposed a systems-based approach for improving adherence to chronic disease therapy. WHO asserts that adherence to treatment is a multidimensional phenomenon governed by the interplay of five sets of factors, also known as "dimensions." These five dimensions include socioeconomic factors such as age, sex, level of family support, and even your type of employment—all of which can affect your ability or willingness to stay on treatment. It also includes patient-related factors, like your knowledge of the disease or perceptions of its risk, condition-related factors, therapy-related factors, and healthcare system–related factors.[30] In other words, how your doctor interacts with you, the amount of follow-up you receive, a medicine's potential side effects, and how you perceive those side effects all impact a patient's willingness to stay on treatment too.

The WHO guidelines are helpful, but words on paper don't help patients. They need to be put into action to address the inevitable adherence challenges every patient will eventually face. Hospitals alone cannot make this happen, and our overreliance on them as the main and only hub for healthcare delivery is getting in the way of patient outcomes. In developed coun-

30 World Health Organization, *Adherence to Long-Term Therapies: Evidence for Action* (Geneva: 2003), http://apps.who.int/iris/bitstream/handle/10665/42682/9241545992.pdf?sequence=1.

tries, the shift in disease burden from acute (appears suddenly and lasts for a short amount of time) to chronic diseases over the past fifty years has rendered acute care models of health service delivery inadequate to address the health needs of the population. In developing countries, this shift is occurring at an even faster rate.

Healthcare policymakers and providers, along with the healthcare institutions they run and work for, need to stop being so insular and open themselves up to other players to support their efforts. In fact, helping patients stay on treatment for as long as they need to actually improve or at least stabilize their condition is bound to have a more significant impact on the health of a population than any single improvement in a single medical treatment ever could. Multidimensional diseases require multi-sectoral, collaborative responses. Just like what we did with the traditional birth attendants to prevent mother-to-child transmission of HIV/AIDS in Tanzania, and with the multi-party models we used to implement VDP, GIPAP, SPAP, Musanda, and others.

Through our work at Axios, it was obvious that getting patients access to an expensive treatment they needed and supporting them to complete their full course of treatment was life-changing at an individual level. But it became obvious that we couldn't ignore the fact that around the world, millions of patients continued to suffer because the root of the issue wasn't being addressed.

We were helping the patients that knocked on our door or at the door of the right physicians, but how about the millions that didn't? Even if treatment suddenly became affordable, free even, or the Jeff Bezoses of the world opened up their coffers to pay for treatment for anyone that needed it, it still would not be enough. We saw it during the HIV epidemic, and then later in the chronic disease patients we managed. Even when treatment was made available, many patients would not be tested or diagnosed early enough, or at all. Others would have no access to a hospital or clinic when they are sick or would stop taking their medications. We had chosen to focus on affordability first given the urgency of the issue, but as we worked with more patients, it was clear it was time to evolve. There was no one there to fill the gap outside the hospital, and we decided, to the extent that we could, to step in. That's why we began looking at more comprehensive programs that helped patients get diagnosed faster, got them access to the treatment they needed, and helped them stay on treatment.

Here's a story from one of our first shared-payment treatment access programs in the UAE. After operating it for a few years, we noticed the average duration of treatment for patients enrolled in the program began to increase. There were several reasons for this. First and foremost, our access programs improved the affordability of treatment making it possible for them to stay on treatment longer and gain better benefits from their treatment. Second, our program managers closely followed up with enrolled patients to ensure they were staying on treatment. They called them whenever it was time to receive another box of medicine and see how they were doing. At the same time, we knew that even if they were getting their treatment at a cost they could afford, to stay on treatment, they would need support to address potential long-term side effects or other physical, psychological, or emotional challenges associated with their disease. After a year and a half, the client came to see us and raised a serious issue. Patients who didn't have such support outside the hospital had a significantly shorter duration of treatment even if their treatment was fully covered or reimbursed. The finding prompted us to look more deeply, and it turns out that it was the personal follow-up that patients received in our programs that was making all the difference. If a call could make such a difference, what could be achieved with other forms of personal support?

Axios developed a tool called the Patient Needs Assessment Tool or PNAT. This tool complemented PFET, the tool I previously told you about that evaluates the financial capacity of the patient to afford the full cost of treatment. PNAT is meant to identify the risk factors that can lead a patient to stop treatment. The results are then used to design a personalized support plan to help the patient stay on treatment. For example, a patient who is found not to be well-informed on the risk of non-adherence receives additional education. Another patient who may have trouble maintaining the proper diet required for successful treatment is partnered with a nutritional coach. Those that just need a daily reminder to take their medicine receive a daily text from one of our program managers. They are simple actions, but they are effective because they are individualized to the needs of the patient.

A published study conducted among patients enrolled in an Axios's patient support program that used PNAT found that a patient's understanding of their disease, involvement in treatment decisions, age, time spent with their physician, and stigma were the factors most likely to affect their ability to stay on treatment. These findings suggest that more emphasis should be placed on meeting patients' information needs, involving them in decisions about their treatment, and allocating sufficient time during medical visits for patients to ask questions. In frequently overburdened healthcare facilities, healthcare professionals are unlikely to have enough time to address all these issues. Other parties must be brought in to complement the work of healthcare professionals and help patients achieve the most from their care and treatment.[31]

Eventually, as we learned and evolved, our shared payment programs for treatment evolved into more comprehensive Patient Support Programs, or PSPs. PSPs brought together multiple parties to offer patients personalized support for diagnosis, access, adherence, and disease monitoring. We soon began conducting PNAT assessments across many of our PSPs. We partnered with psychologists, nutritionists, home care nurses, home delivery specialists, and life coaches, just to name a few. We brought in an entire ecosystem to support patients and close the gap outside the hospital. This ecosystem helped create a critical link between the time the patient exits the hospital and the time they come back in for their follow-up appointment. In return, it improved their ability to manage their disease, their adherence to treatment, and hence their treatment outcome.

When I first left UNAIDS, I knew I wanted to try to do something bold. Something that would change the old, antiquated constructs of how healthcare is provided into a model that actually works for people and makes them healthier and happier. It's been a long road, but project by project, Axios managed to chip away at the dogmatic attitude that has held our health

---

31   Joel Ladner et al., "Factors Impacting Self-Management Ability in Patients with Chronic Diseases in the United Arab Emirates, 2019," *Journal of Comparative Effectiveness Research* 11, no. 3 (February 2022): 179–92, https://doi.org/10.2217/cer-2021-0177.

system back for so long. In the process, we've brought health-care, in a sustainable way, to more than nine million patients in our twenty-five years, and made big headway in changing the mindset of pharmaceutical companies and governments around what is possible.

I learned early on as a boy in war-torn Lebanon that the systems set up to protect us can just as easily fail us. The healthcare system is failing us today. There's no denying it. But the other thing I learned as a young boy is that in times of crisis, you can't wait for someone to give you a solution. You have to put one foot in front of the other and find the solution yourself. That is why I am so proud of what we've been able to accomplish through Axios and its programs. There is even an Access to Medicines Index, run by the Access to Medicines Foundation (ATMF). The ATM Index, as it's known, began as an under-the-radar measurement tool meant to push pharmaceutical companies to act. Thanks to the ATMF director's leadership, and a growing interest in access by pharmaceutical companies, the tool today is pushing the industry toward real change by capturing their progress and shortcomings for the world to see. As investors increasingly turn their focus on companies who are closely linking their business objectives to a broader societal purpose, my hope is that access will only continue to grow as a priority.

In the scope of the world's public health problems, I know that Axios access programs are a drop in the bucket, but they illus-trate the value of a multi-sectoral approach in today's healthcare reality. We have so many examples to back up my theory, and that of many others, that healthcare needs to be more collabo-rative and multi-sectoral. It started with HIV. It continues today with all the work we do at Axios.

It's okay to share the burden. There is no need to silo healthcare by public and private sectors. Healthcare is a public good, as it should be. All of us have a role to play. Without collaboration, healthcare systems cannot improve. We need the public and private sectors, including governments, pharmaceutical companies, providers, hospitals, and third parties like Axios and others to combine our strengths to build more efficient, responsive, and resilient healthcare systems.

It is imperative for countries to look beyond hospitals and tap into complementary, collaborative mechanisms to reach patients wherever they are. Why is it imperative? Why now? Just look at COVID-19. The healthcare system was not capable of managing a global pandemic. Hospitals were bursting at the seams; policymakers shut down their economies in a panic. Why didn't we tap pharmacists or general practitioners to identify and protect the most vulnerable patients, or bring in other parties to create a broader network of facilities to care for sick patients, instead of putting all the burden on hospitals? Because that's not how we've done it in the past. Our physicians too, largely trained in hospitals, develop a very hospital-centric point of view. Many of the health experts advising politicians are physicians themselves and have been raised in this school of thought. That means that when something like COVID-19 comes along, their first instinct is to lock down—as you would in a hospital if a bacteria or virus was identified within its walls. But the real world has many more doors, and you can't shut them all.

At the heart of the problem is the fact that in today's world we often still see hospitals and the healthcare system as one local domestic entity—instead of seeing hospitals and the care provided in that hospital as only a part of a much larger ecosystem in place to keep us healthy. The earliest hospitals in the Middle Ages were the one and only place where people could go for care. That made sense then, but that's not the case in the globalized, hyperconnected world we live in today. Yet we remain overly reliant on hospitals to care for the health of our local communities, cities, and countries. That overreliance on a physical structure has led to an antiquated view of healthcare as a local issue guided by local regulations, maintained by generations of healthcare providers and policymakers educated to believe that this is the only way. It's also a key driver of healthcare gaps and the double standards that we see in healthcare. Today, your life expectancy is completely reliant on the country where you were born.

But there is light at the end of the tunnel. The advent of digital and social technologies have made it easier than ever for us to connect with each other and to bring multiple parties together to support the patient journey. These developments hold incredible promise for healthcare as a whole. But will the healthcare system be willing to adopt them?

Chapter 19

THE GREAT FACILITATOR

Over the last decade, all of us have seen digital technology reshape every aspect of our lives whether we like it or not. But perhaps not surprisingly, healthcare has done a tremendous job of avoiding the digital revolution. If you've ever complained about needing to disconnect from the endless technology-driven chaos of our lives, it's worth asking the healthcare system how they did it. In fact, they've done a fabulous job of staying far, far away from it.

Technology has evolved fast. Very fast. In a little more than forty years, we've gone from computers that used to take up the entire room to palm-sized super-machines, also known as mobile phones, that are smarter than your average adult. These innovations are incredible for many reasons. Of most importance is their ability to facilitate our lives and connect us—to each other, to our possessions, to our bodies. We know more than ever before about our neighbor, the stranger 5,000 miles away, our sleep patterns, our heart rates, the number of steps we take in a day, when our child boarded the bus, when they got off the bus... You get the idea. Unless you are living off the grid, technology—be it our phone, wearables, or social media—is tracking every move you make. It's also given us an endless buffet of tools to reach and connect with each other.

Most industries have happily capitalized on the digitalization of our society. Healthcare, unsurprisingly, has lagged. In a December 2020 interview with *The Economist*, Stephen Klasko, chief executive of Jefferson Health, which runs hospitals in Philadelphia, recounted an exchange he had with a bank executive who told him that twenty years earlier, healthcare and banking were the only industries yet to embrace the consumer and digital revolution. "Now," Mr. Klasko recalls him adding, "you are alone."[32]

Over the last thirty years, other sectors like finance, commerce, and trade managed to break free from local structures and regulations in response to pressures from globalization. A globalized world made them uncomfortable—it created more competition, instability, and a new reality that they didn't know how to navigate. But it also created new financial opportunities that pushed these market-driven sectors to act—and to do so quickly.

Take the finance and commerce sectors, for instance. Before the internet, banking involved visiting your local branch or a trip to the closest ATM. But once personal computers and internet connections became household fixtures, all that changed. It soon became possible to manage your bank account, invest,

---

32 "The Dawn of Digital Medicine," *The Economist*, December 2, 2020, https://www.economist.com/business/2020/12/02/the-dawn-of-digital-medicine.

and make transactions at any time of day from the comfort of your own home. The first bank websites were essentially online brochures. They had product information, photos, contact numbers, and branch maps, but they didn't interact with customers. Soon, banks realized that going online meant less overhead and more profits, some of which could be passed onto consumers in the form of lower fees and better interest rates. Online banking eliminated long lines, reduced waiting times, and made it easier to deliver a more personalized customer experience. As a result, banks prioritized building an online presence. It didn't come without its challenges. At first, people were reluctant to make online payments for security reasons. Then, in 1995, Amazon opened its first online store, offering a much wider selection of products than traditional brick-and-mortar shops. And because it had a significantly lower overhead, prices were cheaper too. Online shopping buoyed confidence in online payments, which in turn led to wider acceptance of online banking services both in Europe and the US.

Today, financial institutions are largely autonomous actors who control money flow and regulate it with little—some might say too little—intervention from the government. Ministries of Finance and central banks largely play a normative role, defining economic and monetary policies to maintain financial stability. It is true that financial institutions didn't necessarily get it right immediately. It has led to excess and mistakes that forced governments to take back some control to manage cash flow. But ultimately it led to change that benefitted the customer. Banks today are mostly virtual and borderless. Currency is the last part of the financial sector that is tied to a specific country. But maybe not for long as cryptocurrency, which functions independently from governments, gains momentum. If it continues to go in that direction, governments may lose the only remaining control mechanism they have in the finance market.

Trade is similar. After the establishment of the World Trade Organization in 1995, whose goal was to ensure that trade flows as smoothly, predictably, and freely as possible, bilateral agreements between countries flourished. While trade barriers do still exist and are used as a political tool from time to time, with support from a globalized financial system, we are increasingly moving toward free trade between countries. Supply shortages faced by the UK post-Brexit are perfect examples of why a borderless trade system is best. Truck drivers don't even want to go to the UK anymore because they must wait long hours at the border and earn less money.

The supply chain has also become largely borderless, a development facilitated by a globalized financial and trade system. This became an important issue with COVID-19 when countries closed up. Even two years later, the supply chain hasn't recovered yet, highlighting the conflict that exists between our globalized world and hyperlocal healthcare decision-making.

Even your local restaurants have adapted. Restaurants, much like hospitals, used to rely solely on their physical structure and the people inside that structure—the chef, the waiter, the host. If you were hungry and didn't want to cook at home, it used to be that your only option was to go to a physical restaurant and be served your chef-prepared food by a waiter. Globalization created more competition for local restaurants as the ease of obtaining new, even foreign ingredients led to a bigger variety of offerings in cities around the world. Plus, as customers became more accustomed to virtual banking, shopping online, and other conveniences, they began to crave convenience in their food too. From that was born the booming food delivery business we rely on today.

The truth is that healthcare today is a sector in direct conflict with our globalized world. While science and medicine have evolved at an unprecedented pace thanks to recent technological advancements, the same can't be said for the mechanisms that exist to deliver that care and treatment to patients. Here's a mind-blowing statistic to give you an idea of how right that bank executive was: around 70 percent of American hospitals still fax and mail patient records. In France, it is even more, almost all.

It's hard to imagine how the healthcare system has managed to stay so antiquated. Well, we know the reason—it's because the healthcare system is largely seen as a domestic service for the local community. Isn't that what a hospital is all about? And isn't the hospital and healthcare system seen, unnecessarily, as one? But even knowing why, it's hard to comprehend how we let healthcare—such an important part of a functioning society— get so far behind. If we, as humans, refused to use a computer or a cellphone, we'd be cut off from the majority of jobs and many of our relationships and social connections. However, the insular, siloed nature of our healthcare infrastructure has made it possible for our system to continue with business as usual despite the incredible shifts going on around it.

Any evolution that has taken place within our healthcare system has mostly been kept at a facility level—no surprise given the overreliance on hospitals and the hyperlocal focus of the health-care system. Some hospitals digitize their patient files, and have online portals where patients can schedule appointments, see test results, and email their doctors—but that information starts and ends at the hospital. It's not being shared with other parties that could benefit from that information or scaled up to a health system level.

Essentially, the world's current digital health infrastructure is made up of millions of one-off digital interfaces that don't talk to each other. And that has a huge impact on patient outcomes. For example, you go to your doctor because you are feeling sick. She enters all your information, symptoms, and prescribed treatment in her hospital system. You start taking your medication and it makes you feel terrible so you stop taking it and it makes you feel even worse. You can't get an appointment with her fast enough because she's booked for months, so you go to an urgent care center not affiliated with the hospital. That urgent care center is fully reliant on you to tell them your medical history and what you were prescribed because they don't have any of the information your doctor captured available to them. If you don't know what medication you were prescribed, you can find yourself walking out of urgent care with the same prescription that made you feel bad in the first place. That may result in an even more serious reaction or worse. The COVID-19 pandemic made many of these issues obvious. The nonexistent or, at best, incoherent healthcare digital infrastructure meant that we couldn't reach patients when we needed to. We also couldn't fully track vaccinations and outcomes, making post-safety surveillance much harder and lengthier than it needed to be. And that's just the tip of the iceberg.

Data security and patient confidentiality are often painted as the major barriers to digitalization in healthcare. While important, we already know how to overcome this issue. At this stage, it's just a comfortable scapegoat for a much less public relations–friendly reason. Why is our health information more protected than our finances? Or our personal social media information? The artificial barriers erected around data sharing and the hesitancy to build more collaborative digital platforms are largely driven by a resistance to decentralizing care. Decentralizing care means money lost by hospitals because patients will become less tied to one institution. It also threatens the precious doctor–patient relationship. That relationship is critical. I know that firsthand. Yet there's a way to preserve that relationship, even foster it, through digital interventions that help reinforce important patient–doctor discussions. Technology has the potential to completely change how we care for patients. I'd argue healthcare is the industry that has the most to gain from digitalization. Yet healthcare decision-makers and hospitals are so stuck in their ways that they're standing in the way of the very thing they swore to protect.

If you think about it, most of the hospital-level innovation we see today is based on the concept of patients going to the hospital, not the other way round. These tools provide a means for a patient to look into the service they received at the hospital or plan to receive in the future. But what if we had digital tools that allowed them to connect with their patients, check in on how they were doing, interact with them, and even virtually monitor their performance on treatment outside the hospital? And what if these tools were built in collaboration with partners outside the hospital that could support doctors to achieve the best for their patient? The impact on patients would be life-changing. Even more for those living with chronic conditions where follow-up is a make or break.

Patients today are more informed and engaged in their health than ever before. They have the entire internet at their disposal to help them understand how they are feeling. Many, especially younger patients of forty and under—have lived the majority of their lives with technology. They are used to being connected. To having information easily at their disposal. To making appointments with a simple click. Getting in touch with anyone they want to with a two-second text message. The only part of their lives that remains disconnected is perhaps the most important one—their health.

At a patient level, digital tools can empower patients, helping them understand their disease and their full treatment journey. We know that the more informed a patient is, the better they do. Countless research has shown that, including the latest research on Axios's adherence tool that I mentioned to you earlier, which found that patients with a stronger understanding of their disease are more likely to be able to self-manage their chronic conditions.

At a system level, digital tools have the potential to facilitate multidimensional, collaborative care and treatment. They are the perfect antidote to fill the gap outside the hospital that I discussed in the previous chapter. At Axios, we are running our own system to do just that across our support programs in hopes that it can one day be replicated and scaled up to help patients at a much broader scale. The digital tools we developed, including mobile apps and online interfaces, are designed to improve the medical outcomes of treatment by facilitating the connections between those who make treatment access possible across our programs. That includes Axios program managers, patients, physicians, pharmacists, and in some cases, charities.

While they are Axios-owned tools, they are directly integrated within pharmacy systems. Unidentified information is appropriately shared to ensure every party involved in helping that patient achieve success has the information they need to make important decisions. For example, using these tools, we've been able to personalize and improve our own patient support programs by more easily and more quickly identifying trends in treatment use, and the factors getting in the way of their treatment. During COVID-19, the same tools were used to connect with our most vulnerable patients to make sure they continued to receive their treatment despite not being able to go to the hospital.

We see these tools as facilitators, not replacements for human connection. This is an important distinction for me. Digital is often painted as the be-all and end-all solution to the world's problems. I don't see it that way. Human connection will forever be at the heart of how healthcare is practiced. Digital tools will never replace that, but they can certainly help simplify and facilitate connected care by creating a simpler, more convenient link between providers and receivers of healthcare.

I'll admit that, much like the healthcare system as a whole, Axios was slow to integrate digital tools into how we work with patients. The digital world is so far removed from the day-to-day of healthcare delivery that it's easy to forget that there exists this huge, largely untapped set of tools at our disposal to help us better support patients. We still have a lot of work to do, but our small successes have given us a taste of the significant potential of digital technologies to transform healthcare, much like they did in finance, trade, and retail.

We can't talk about digital technology and ignore social media.

It, too, has a critical role to play in improving health outcomes. Through social media, we now have platforms that can reach the entire world with a health message in a click.

Take a second to think about how powerful that is. Unfortunately, as we know well, that power hasn't always been used for good. The level of misinformation across social media platforms related to the COVID-19 pandemic prompted WHO to brand it an "infodemic," or when too much information, including false or misleading information, exists in digital and physical environments during a disease outbreak. This infodemic was incredibly detrimental to our global COVID-19 response. The loudest voices won out over reason and science time and time again, and credible facts were pushed down and dismissed. It caused confusion, prompted mistrust in health authorities, and undermined the public health response. That is very dangerous. During COVID-19, people drank bleach, took medicines meant to prevent parasites in animals, and even believed that the COVID-19 vaccines were outfitted with microchips in an evil plot by Microsoft's Bill Gates to control the world. It sounds like a joke, and perhaps many of us thought this kind of misinformation would never reach the levels that it did, but we miscalculated.

To make things worse, social media algorithms are being adjusted to only show you the kind of content you like (because why would you come back to the platform to see a bunch of people talking about something you don't agree with?). Over time, if you keep seeing the same information, true or not, posted over and over by people you love or respect, you'll believe it. It's just human nature.

By leaving social media unchecked for so long, we've allowed an entirely new, false reality to be created. In this wild west of social media, every word you say is held up to the court of public opinion. There's nothing inherently wrong with that. It's important to be pushed to back up your beliefs and to think differently than the masses. But moderation is needed. Once a photo or thought is posted on social media, it instantly becomes fodder for judgment. In a matter of seconds, it enters the global narrative and what we collectively understand to be real and true—despite the fact that it may be quite unreal or quite untrue. Yet what's happening today is that those with the most outlandish thoughts and with the least authority to be saying anything of substance at all are the ones doing all—or most—of the talking on social media.

Those with more reasonable points of view are growing tired of it all, leaving behind an ever-growing narrative of false information that is affecting what we believe and how we judge fact from fiction. The most sensible, evidence-based voices are being overwhelmed by those that talk the loudest, leaving behind a critical mass of incorrect health information that is influencing political decisions and interrupting critical public health response.

Once again, healthcare's inability to adjust to the digital landscape severely limited our ability to respond to the COVID-19 pandemic. Digital tools could have been used to target our prevention efforts by more easily identifying the most vulnerable before they ever got sick. Similarly, social media, without a unified scientific voice and proper governance, turned into a machine for misinformation instead of an incredible platform to disseminate consistent health information to the whole world at the click of a button.

Technology isn't going anywhere. In fact, it stands to play a critical role in addressing many of the gaps we've discussed in this book by serving as the great facilitator. People will always be at the center of quality care because medicine is not black and white. Quality care is personalized care. We need doctors and nurses that have the time to actually talk to their patients and follow up on their progress. Digital tools can help minimize the burden on their time and close the gap outside the hospital so they have more opportunities to connect with patients, virtually or in person. There is no shortage of mobile apps and digital tools that are designed to do just what I've laid out here. What we don't currently have is a flexibility on the part of public health stakeholders to accept a new way of doing things and a willingness to invest in scaling these new solutions for the greater good.

The forces of technology are now deep and strong in our society. Whether we like it or not, technology is ingrained in our day-to-day lives, driving many of our actions, decisions, and thoughts. There is no avoiding it. Eventually, healthcare will no longer have the choice to look away.

Chapter 20

IT'S TIME WE MOVE FORWARD

Public health, or health in general, has the potential to turn our lives upside down. Most of us only realize that when we or a family member gets sick. COVID-19, even for the lucky ones, brought that reality to each of our doorsteps. I feel that today we are in the midst of a critical intersection and it's up to us to make sure we learn the lessons presented to us and build a better system than what we started with.

I know the story I've told you wasn't always a pretty one, but I felt it was important to revisit how the world reacted to HIV and how much that changed today with COVID-19. Along the way, I hope I've connected some of the dots to illustrate the widening gap between the traditional role of the hospital and the changing needs of patients. This widening gap requires an overhaul of the healthcare system, not more hospitals and more of the same. Paradoxically, more globalized healthcare will lead to better individual patient care.

We've covered a lot of ground. I want to make sure all of you reading this book walk away with a clear understanding of why healthcare is not doing what we want it to do. So, in summary, here it is.

Our politicians, policymakers, healthcare professionals, medical schools, and many others in the healthcare field perceive healthcare as a local, community issue, putting entirely too much focus on the hospital as the center of that system. This unnecessary hyper-localized focus makes the healthcare system a hostage to geopolitics. Geopolitics is a word that's thrown around a lot and can mean a lot of things. I define it as the way a country's size, position, and other factors can directly or indirectly influence its power and its relationships with other countries.

Following the 2008 global economic crisis, our world turned inward, creating an entirely different geopolitical environment than we had during our HIV response. We saw the devastation that can come from interconnected, globalized financial systems, and politicians capitalized on the opportunity to preach a new brand of nationalism and populism that threatened the new world order that had flourished since the end of the Cold War. This period is looking increasingly similar to the post-1929 recession that led to World War II. Would-be-authoritarian leaders like Donald Trump in the United States broke away from major global deals like the Paris Climate Agreement, preaching that these deals were against the best interest of the United States. Brexit led to the divorce of the United Kingdom and

Europe. China became increasingly insular. Russia stepped up its campaign to challenge democratic principles, weaken its opponents, and waged war on Ukraine.

These are just a few examples of geopolitical changes that weakened our democracies and our healthcare response. During COVID-19, this new reality encouraged public distrust in reliable scientific sources, preventing a unified scientific voice. They weakened the mandates of supranational bodies like WHO, giving them little power to oversee or enforce any one clear path. They also pushed for pointless border-centric solutions, like lockdowns, instead of more effective global solutions. Not once did the world's ministers of health come together to craft a unified response against COVID-19. Everyone chose to do their own thing. We saw as many policies, often contradictory, as there are countries. Each country put in place often baseless rules and regulations that tried to contain viruses within their borders—yet globalization is inherent to every aspect of society. That is why these measures did little to stop the pandemic, and in some cases, only fueled it. It's no surprise that country responses, for the most part, weren't successful. We were far from the globalized world of the 1990s.

Today's geopolitical environment is unnecessarily locking healthcare inside domestic borders. This translates to an aversion to collaboration, an overfocus on local hospitals and clinics as the only source of healthcare delivery, and a reinforcement of the inflexible tendencies of the healthcare system. COVID-19 put all of these issues on display for the entire world to see.

So are we destined for inadequate healthcare forever? In our current geopolitical environment, I have no doubt that government leaders will continue to hide behind their borders in the short term. They'll implement new rules and regulations to limit other players and to maintain their power. Yet I believe these defense mechanisms will fade over time when the dire long-term economic, social, and medical consequences of insular politics come to fruition. There is a gap and new players will undoubtedly fill the void. As powers shift, our borders will become more fluid, making country-level laws and regulations less relevant and less restrictive.

Why do we need so many national laws and regulations when our challenges and their solutions are increasingly global? The social and economic influence of the digital technology industry will push us forward as well. I predict that the tension between global health threats (like COVID-19 and future pandemics), global technology, and an antiquated, localized healthcare mindset is what will ultimately push us forward. Globalization is bound to prevail, and with it, democratic principles of openness, tolerance, and freedom. There is no turning back, and even if we face some digression, it will be temporary. Although it may not seem like it right now, it's simply human nature. We first built shelter in caves. Then we went to small villages and eventually to cities. We never went back. We've built a global village and have benefitted as a result, and despite the ups and downs that we may face, we'll continue a forward trajectory. At this point, we are all dependent on globalization. We can't have globalization without democratic principles, and we can't innovate and move forward without collaboration.

Ultimately, globalized healthcare is better healthcare. Imagine a world where you'd have access to not just the doctors in your backyard, but the best doctors in the world right at your fingertips, or highly specialized doctors who may not exist in your city through telemedicine. Market dynamics would drive service improvements and capacity building in the medical field, helping to standardize healthcare and ultimately bringing more quality care to a much bigger portion of the population. Patients could have access to personalized support at the push of a button. Critical medicines, not held back by local regulations, would be available more readily, equitably, and perhaps less expensively too. One country may not have the volume of patients to make a price reduction worth it for pharmaceutical or medical supply companies, but if companies saw the world as their marketplace, the sheer volume would make price reductions much more feasible. Minimizing our overreliance on hospitals, which account for a significant portion of healthcare spending in all countries, will also bring costs down for patients. And of course, globalizing healthcare will help make it less vulnerable to geopolitical factors—minimizing, if not avoiding, many of the challenges and consequences we experienced during COVID-19. While in many cases you may still need to receive care locally, the care provided would be improved and optimized through a globalized healthcare system.

This concept is much like your dinner delivery order. It may be cooked locally, but using ingredients from around the world makes it taste even better. A local delivery driver brings it directly to you in thirty minutes, thanks to the infrastructure built to support digital apps like Uber Eats, Deliveroo, and others. If only we could flip a switch and apply the same principles to healthcare.

Instead, an unnecessarily solely localized healthcare system that is overly reliant on local hospitals and resistant to change is creating a perilous world, unable to respond to emerging diseases, global health threats, and emergencies. The world has changed and so must healthcare.

Take the typical patient journey. Patients are mobile these days. They have the internet. The patient experience no longer needs to be restricted to a local hospital the same way it was in the Middle Ages. It is important to see your local doctor when you need in-person care, but it shouldn't be your only option. Local care will always be essential, but it's no longer enough. If you are dealing with a serious or unique condition, your local doctor may not have the experience to treat you. Plus, as populations grow and pandemics prevail, cities will no longer be able to care for their population within hospital walls. How many hospitals can you build in one city? And why should you? We will have no choice but to fill the space outside the hospital with complementary players unless we want to leave patients behind.

If globalized healthcare is where we are headed, how do we get there?

In the short term, I see the private sector stepping up to fill the gaps that have come to the surface during COVID-19, just like they did in my stories about prevention of mother-to-child transmission of HIV/AIDS, cancer treatment access, and most recently in the shared-payment programs we do at Axios. And just like they did in the digital, banking, and trade industries when they were forced to adapt to a new globalized world. They have a financial incentive to do so. The COVID-19 vaccine is a great example of a major gap they were able to fill—and fast. If we relied on the government to develop the vaccine, we'd be waiting for years. They also already have access to the digital tools and resources we need to fill the space outside the hospital and better support patients when they get sick. All they need are laws and regulations that incentivize non-public stakeholders to scale their innovation for the greater good.

We don't need governments to step up and solve all our problems alone. We just need them to open the door to multi-stakeholder collaboration. Even if governments were to suddenly get their act together, it won't be enough. Even when good things happen at the top—like US President Obama's Affordable Care Act, for example—it doesn't trickle down sufficiently to result in systemic change because the system itself is broken. Private sector interventions alone won't be enough either. To fix the major healthcare gaps we face today, we need bottom-up solutions, and we need multiple actors to participate, just like what we did with Axios's access programs.

Remember what happened in the UAE with the Dubai Health Authority? When a government spearheads the efforts and mobilizes relevant public and private stakeholders, change happens quickly and the effects trickle down just as quickly to patients and other end users. Those programs are a drop in the bucket in comparison to the scale of the immense public health challenges we face today, but they do show us what works and what is possible when multiple parties—public, private, and otherwise—come together to achieve a common goal.

A More Effective Healthcare System Closes the Gap Outside the Hospital

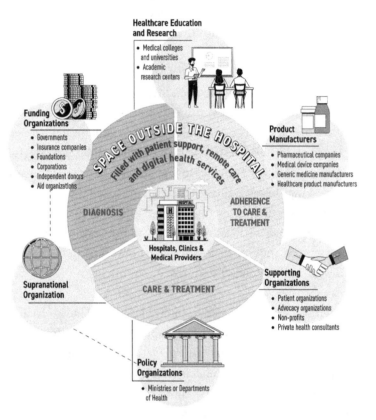

Healthcare Education and Research
- Medical colleges and universities
- Academic research centers

Funding Organizations
- Governments
- Insurance companies
- Foundations
- Corporations
- Independent donors
- Aid organizations

Product Manufacturers
- Pharmaceutical companies
- Medical device companies
- Generic medicine manufacturers
- Healthcare product manufacturers

SPACE OUTSIDE THE HOSPITAL
Filled with patient support, remote care and digital health services

DIAGNOSIS

ADHERENCE TO CARE & TREATMENT

Hospitals, Clinics & Medical Providers

CARE & TREATMENT

Supranational Organization

Supporting Organizations
- Patient organizations
- Advocacy organizations
- Non-profits
- Private health consultants

Policy Organizations
- Ministries or Departments of Health

Much of healthcare happens outside a hospital or health facility. That is why a more effective healthcare system invites other parties to complement hospitals and clinics to provide patients with more comprehensive support.

This brings us to an important point: governance. If healthcare is globalized, with multiple parties from around the world contributing, how do we set standards and maintain and monitor the quality of the care and treatment being provided? Globalized healthcare will require a governance structure that is forward-thinking and responsive to the needs of its people yet driven by evidence and not reelection. I think we can all agree on that. But if not country governments alone, who should establish the rules and who should enforce them?

Globalized healthcare, like finance and trade, will require supranational oversight and international laws and regulations. As they stand today, United Nations agencies, like the World Health Organization, are not adequate for such a role. These groups have been significantly affected by the digital revolution and geopolitical shifts. The current geopolitical environment has whittled down their role to a largely normative one since the HIV days. They provide recommendations and guidance but have little to no power to implement or enforce them. To address these issues, there have been recent efforts to improve WHO's funding and governance model and to increase funding overall, but that will not be enough. A change in their mandate is what is really needed, and could have been helpful during COVID-19. Yet such a change would require agreement and investment by its member countries and the world of 2020 was simply not interested in a major global body telling them what to do within their own borders. This kind of consensus may be difficult to achieve in today's world. In this case, an alternative supranational body could take the shape of groups like the G7, the G20, or the European Commission. These groups, which have proven successful in providing oversight to the trade and finance sectors, work by creating a unified position across key countries with the expectation that other countries will then follow. To achieve the level of collaboration that is needed in healthcare, however, such a governance model would need to convene players from multiple sectors, not just public sector leaders.

Borderless topics need borderless oversight. An adequate

supranational oversight body for healthcare should go beyond national politics, encourage collaboration, and bring harmony to globalized care by setting consistent international standards and ensuring that those standards are followed by all involved parties. These standards would serve as drivers of a unified, consistent scientific voice, which, as you now know well from this book, is imperative to better healthcare. With the barrage of information we now all receive on a daily basis, a unified scientific voice needs to be louder and clearer than ever. It may not be possible to offset all the noise generated in social media, but it will provide a credible and coherent alternative message to help rebuild public trust.

Supranational standards would also serve as guidance for individual communities. This is an important point to pause on. Globalized healthcare doesn't mean local, community-level healthcare disappears. As I said before, the nature of healthcare delivery will mean that your local doctor, hospital, clinic, or pharmacy will always have an important role to play in providing you with in-person care. In globalized healthcare, these local providers of care would follow globalized standards, but would still be free, with the support of local policymakers, to customize services to the needs of their particular community.

We should also ask ourselves whether social media, given its incredible reach, could play this role with proper oversight. Or perhaps we should ask ourselves whether it already does. Twitter had the power to shut down the President of the United States when it deleted Trump's account in 2020. Whether you think that's a good or bad thing, we can't deny its impact or value as a mechanism that makes it possible to reach nearly the entire world through one platform. There is no other mechanism in the world like that. It's incredibly powerful, and as with all powerful forces, they can be manifested in both good and bad ways.

There will always be negative voices, but I truly believe that if we can start to show the world that better healthcare is possible, the court of public opinion will come together to overcome the naysayers and deniers and demand better. It won't just be a group of standalone advocates shouting for change and struggling to get attention. Through social media, we'll have an entire global army pushing us forward. Obviously, if social media is to play this role moving forward, we need significantly more investment in identifying ways to monitor and provide guidelines to this new world—starting first by balancing its profit motive and adjusting its algorithm so that it's more reflective of a balanced global dialogue.

Social media today is quite the paradox—on one end, it's a platform that is connecting humans in an unprecedented way, creating a common reality that has the potential to create a new kind of conscientious, responsive, and more equitable society. On the other hand, it's slowly chipping away at many of the democratic ideals the world has suffered so much to build.

Here's a prime example. Social media is making it hard for leaders—within and outside the government—to do anything significant. Anyone in the public spotlight in a leadership position is judged so harshly by the court of public opinion on social media for every word they say that they are scared of doing anything at all. This is what I call the principle of precaution. But just because a decision is unpopular doesn't mean it's bad. What is bad is stagnation and making no decision at all.

Growing fragmentation and double standards in our society have led to a crisis where everyone is continuously trying to find someone to blame, and social media has only magnified the issue. It's important that our elected officials, business leaders, and others in positions of power are held accountable, but not to the extent that they are immobilized. During COVID-19, we saw politicians waffle back and forth in fear of offending their constituents for not doing enough, or doing too much. Every week, citizens received different directions about how to prevent COVID-19. Local rules and regulations changed almost daily. The public was confused to the point where trust was lost. At a time when we needed leadership more than ever, our leaders were afraid to lead. COVID-19 is a perfect example of what can happen when democratic principles are put to the test. When our leaders are no longer allowed to make mistakes, they will no longer make decisions. Without decisions and leadership, we can't have change. Without change, there is no evolution—and healthcare needs to evolve.

Ultimately, it's individuals that change the world. Healthcare will be "fixed" by innovative leaders willing to take risks and do things differently. In my opinion, we need to look beyond those educated under an antiquated medical curriculum for leadership. I believe the future of healthcare is likely to be driven by leaders outside the healthcare space applying what they learned in other industries. Much of what I've been able to accomplish in access over the last thirty years has happened because of individuals who were willing to think and act outside the box. Throughout the twentieth century, leaders used aggression and stubbornness to dominate their opposition, condemning vulnerability and understanding as signs of weakness. There are still plenty of leaders like that today, but this archetype of the strongman is being challenged by a new generation of leaders that come from a variety of races and genders and believe that leadership comes from raising people up, not keeping them down. We need these forward-thinking actors—at an international, national, and local level—to help accelerate the transformation we need in healthcare. And all of us have a role to play in raising up these unconventional voices.

In healthcare, more people living in the world means fewer resources to go around. Medicines, with the upcoming shift to personalized medications, stand to become even costlier. Universal healthcare has given many in poorer countries access to the basics but also triggered patients to ask for more. Double standards are a fact of life and will only continue to grow. Throughout my career in access to healthcare, the hardest lesson I've had to learn is that providing equal access to all is utopia. But that doesn't mean it's pointless. What we can do is find solutions to reduce the gaps and improve our standards by mobilizing a health system designed to make our world healthier, not sicker.

While it may not be possible to bring the same standard of quality healthcare to every human on Earth, at the population level, globalized healthcare will significantly improve access to healthcare overall. In the end, we are looking for *better* care for all, even if we can't achieve the *same* care for all. The implications of not adapting healthcare to our new world are clear as day for any of us who lived through the COVID-19 pandemic. We no longer have a choice to sit back and ride the status quo. We owe it to our children and future generations.

In the end, I do believe that the future of healthcare is a brighter one. We will get there driven by motivated private companies and civil society, public–private collaboration, a growing chorus of voices demanding change, and a new generation of leaders willing to try something new. Social media and digital technologies will shift healthcare-seeking behavior beyond conventional patient–doctor models. Individuals and communities will be keen to exchange information, tools, and best practices and to experience a more collaborative world facilitated by the digital revolution. With these forces at work, healthcare will eventually open up to globalization and break free from geopolitical forces. It will be a bumpy road. No change comes without challenge. Traditional healthcare actors will continue to push for business as usual. Pharmaceutical companies will continue to resist new treatment access models. Politicians will fight to keep their hold on healthcare in an effort to keep their power. I hope it will not take several pandemics like COVID-19 to complete the transformation.

Although I've always been labeled as much more of a skeptic than an optimist, I am cautiously optimistic. COVID-19 opened the world's eyes to the gaps in the healthcare system and the implications of this negligence. Millions of people have died from HIV/AIDS and COVID-19 and continue to every day. We can't let their deaths be for nothing. We have to fill the gaps in the healthcare system, and we will. Nature doesn't like a void. Humans, from our earliest days as *Homo sapiens*, have a unique cognitive ability to analyze and adapt. We will find a way. My vision has always been about initiating momentum and making small but critical moves to inspire big changes. I will continue to do that in whatever way I can through Axios and by sharing my story and what I've learned along the way.

In the last century, healthcare has become somewhat of a dirty word. It's associated with political battles, cutthroat insurance companies nickel-and-diming you when you need care most, greedy pharmaceutical companies, and countless examples of system failure—from COVID-19 to maternal health to the millions of people around the world who don't have access to even basic medicines. That sentiment is a dangerous one because it pushes people away, including the people we need to help make it better. Healthcare is a human right. It's something we all need and deserve. It's something that impacts every single piece of our lives. Without our health, we have nothing. I can't think of anything more worth fighting for. It's time we finally got it right.

ACKNOWLEDGMENTS

Anne Reeler, my friend and partner at Axios, once told me: "You are like a sponge, you absorb all the information you are given." From a young age, I was curious about almost everything. I listened and watched all that came my way to understand and learn. I watched the mechanic who repaired my father's car, the electrician, the plumber, my best friend's father, the university lecturer... I could go on and on. This has never changed until now.

I am very thankful for all those in my life who have fed my curiosity and taught me so much. The list of my acknowledgments would be too long if I included all the people who helped me progress in the journey I described in this book. I apologize to those who have not been listed or whom I may have omitted inadvertently.

Marie-Helene, my wife, has unwaveringly supported me every step of the way, through the good and the bad. She was never afraid of the unknown and always willing to explore new frontiers. I wouldn't have been who I am today without her. Thank you for always being by my side.

Thank you to my children, Jean-Noel, Eliott, and Paul, who stayed by my side despite my frequent travels. They often spent weeks without seeing me. Today, I am so proud of who they've become.

My parents, Jean and Georgette, who gave me endless love and who didn't spare any sacrifice to give me the best education that opened the doors for me. And my sister Salma for her love and care.

I want to thank Professor Chapman, who opened his department and his arms when I left Lebanon to come to France. When I asked him why he picked me among so many others without ever meeting me, he said: "When I read your letter, you basically wanted me to give you a shot. So I did." Thank you for helping me start my new life and integrate into French society.

Thank you also to Professor Vildé, my mentor who helped me immensely to grow as a professional and backed me up when I decided to join the World Health Organization. You were always so committed to helping your students find the best opportunities. A true professor.

I can't forget Jose Esparza, who opened the door for me at the World Health Organization, welcomed me into his team, taught me diplomacy, and helped me to see the world with a different lens.

I also need to mention Anne Winter, who offered unlimited

support during a very difficult time when UNAIDS was under attack, and David Corkery, who taught me to be a spokesperson and who remains a dear friend and counselor.

I want to thank my partners and co-founders of Axios, Anne Reeler, Brian Elliott, John Macdonald, Peter Ahern, and Sowedi Muyingo, who, like me, made the leap into the unknown. With faith, courage, and resilience, it paid off.

To Anas Nofal, Roshel Jayasundera, and Cliona Brady, the new generation of colleagues and partners who share my passion and took Axios and its solutions to a whole new level. I am grateful to you and very proud of what you have done and are continuing to do.

Last but not least, thank you Mariana Rodrigues for helping me to create a stronger Axios brand and to communicate my passion over the past ten years. And, of course, thank you for helping me write this book. Nobody, not even me, could have expressed what I felt better than you did.

These acknowledgments wouldn't be complete without mentioning my childhood friends who accompanied my journey from the onset:

Mosbah El Khatib, my friend for as long as I can remember. We grew up together. I learned from you to sometimes see life from a different angle. This helped me in my journey and in this book. Thank you for such a meaningful friendship.

Najib Lyan, my cousin and my dear caring childhood friend, and my lawyer. Thank you for a very rich friendship and for helping me structure Axios with the highest international standards.

Said Saouma, whom I met during my first residency. You've been by my side since we moved to France from Lebanon and you've become like family since.

ABOUT THE AUTHOR

JOSEPH SABA, MD, is an infectious disease physician working on the frontline of access to healthcare since the early days of the HIV/AIDS pandemic.

Throughout his career, Joseph has led numerous discussions with pharmaceutical companies, governments, and other key players across the healthcare community to drive access to innovative medications in low- and middle-income countries (LMICs). He is known internationally for establishing the first antiretroviral drug access program through the UNAIDS Drug Access Initiative, making it possible for critical medicines to reach patients in need during the peak of the HIV/AIDS epidemic and pioneering a new generation of treatment access solutions for LMICs.

In 1993, Joseph joined the World Health Organization (WHO) as the WHO Focal Point for the National Plan for HIV Vaccine Development. From 1994–1995, he worked with the WHO Global Program on AIDS in Rwanda and later supported HIV vaccine research efforts in Geneva. Following his time at WHO, he worked at the Joint United Nations Program on HIV/AIDS in the Department of Policy, Strategy, and Research, where he led a global research effort focused on the prevention of mother-to-child transmission (PMTCT) of HIV/AIDS, as well as the groundbreaking PETRA study, a multicenter clinical trial on PMTCT treatment in Africa.

For the last twenty-three years, Joseph has served as the CEO of Axios International, a healthcare access company he co-founded, which has developed programs to improve patient access to healthcare in more than one hundred countries.

He completed his medical degree at St. Joseph University (Beirut, Lebanon) and his infectious diseases specialty, along with a certificate of medical statistics, at the University Paris VI (France). Joseph also holds a master's in communications and medical management (MSc) from the Superior Business School (Paris, France). He is fluent in Arabic, French, and English.

Joseph has been featured in the *Wall Street Journal*, *International Herald Tribune*, *Newsweek*, and *Pharmaceutical Executive*, among others, and has been published widely in peer-reviewed scientific journals.

For more information, media requests, and speaking engagements, visit joseph-saba.com.

CPSIA information can be obtained
at www.ICGtesting.com
Printed in the USA
BVHW030944080323
659891BV00015B/751/J

9 781544 535289